SECRETS OF
TANTRIC SEX

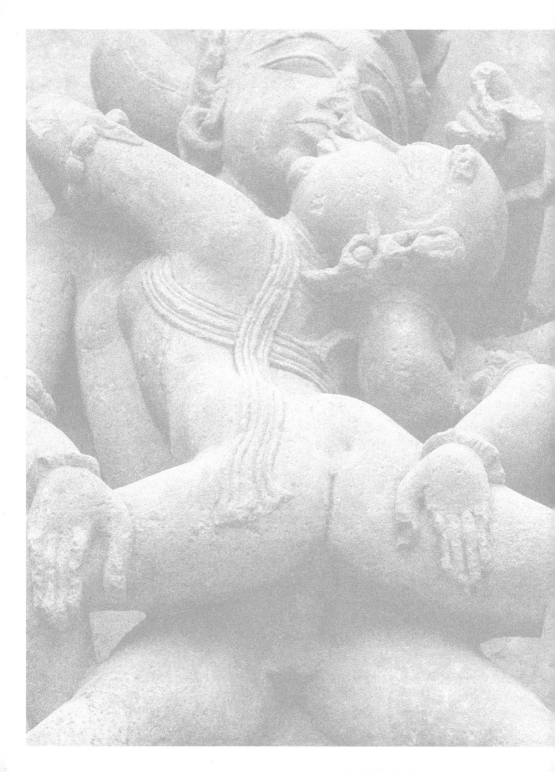

SECRETS OF
TANTRIC SEX

CLAUDIA BLAKE

IVY PRESS

First published in the UK in 2018 by
Ivy Press
An imprint of The Quarto Group
The Old Brewery, 6 Blundell Street
London N7 9BH, United Kingdom
T (0)20 7700 6700 F (0)20 7700 8066
www.QuartoKnows.com

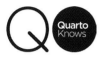

British Library Cataloguing-in-Publication Data
A catalogue record for this book is available from the British Library

ISBN: 978-1-78240-575-7

This book was conceived, designed and produced by
Ivy Press
58 West Street, Brighton, BN1 2RA, United Kingdom

Publisher: Susan Kelly
Creative Director: Michael Whitehead
Design & Art Direction: Wayne Blades, Kevin Knight
Editorial Director: Tom Kitch
Project Editor: Caroline Earle
Photographer: Neal Grundy
Illustrations: Nicky Ackland-Snow, Peters & Zabransky
Assistant Editor: Jenny Campbell
Tantric Consultant: Bryony Henderson
Models: Bryony Henderson, Luke Lambert
Make-up Artists: Justine Rice, Bella Hamilton

Cover image: Shutterstock/Grinnum

Printed by GPS Group

10 9 8 7 6 5 4 3 2

Note from the publisher

Although every effort has been made to ensure that the information
presented in this book is correct, the authors and publisher cannot
be held responsible for any injuries that may arise.

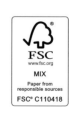

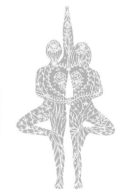

FSC
www.fsc.org
MIX
Paper from
responsible sources
FSC® C110418

How to Use This Book   6
Introduction   8

Chapter 1: **Preparing the Spirit**   **16**

Chapter 2: **Preparing the Body**   **52**

Chapter 3: **Preparing the Partnership**   **86**

Chapter 4: **Drawing Close**   **124**

Chapter 5: **Exploring Ecstasies**   **156**

Chapter 6: **Deep in Pleasure**   **188**

Appendices
Glossary   216
Further Reading   218
Web Sites   219
Index   220
Acknowledgments   224

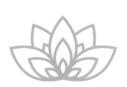
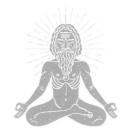
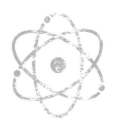

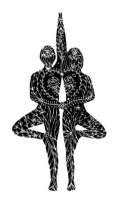

Harmony

The Tantric couple doesn't have to be perfect—just willing to give ourselves to the experience and enjoy what comes. Harmony doesn't mean perfection: it just means we move together.

HOW TO USE THIS BOOK

This book is intended as an introductory guide for those interested in exploring the delights of Tantric lovemaking. Tantra is an ancient and complex tradition, and if you want to look into it as a religion, there are many books and teachers: this is a book for lovers eager to put a first toe into the deep waters. It is divided into five chapters, beginning with meditation and sensuality practices you can do by yourself, and then moving on to ways you can use Tantra to enrich your sex life with a partner. While you can dip in and out, it is recommended you read the chapters in order.

Important Notice

When it comes to lovemaking, safety—both emotional and physical—is the foundation of any ethical relationship, Tantric or otherwise. Tantra was created in the days long before safe sex, but that's no reason not to practice it now. Unless you and your partner are absolutely sure there's no risk, always use condoms and pay good attention to birth control. There's nothing unspiritual or unromantic about making sure sex brings only pleasure instead of problems—quite the opposite!

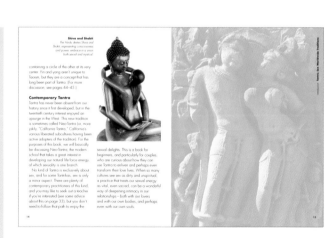

Background

The introductory section of this book looks at the history of Tantra in the context of worldwide religion.

Understanding Ecstasy

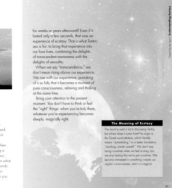

Feel the moment
When we are gladly present in the moment, any experience can become ecstatic.

If you start studying Tantric sex, you'll hear the word "ecstasy" mentioned a lot. It sounds wonderful – but what, in this context, does it actually mean?

Human beings are experience-seekers, and yet experiences can often leave us feeling a little flat. A rollercoaster gives us a rush of adrenaline, and for a short time we're euphoric, but after a while the feeling settles down and we start to want more. A delicious meal is comforting, but once it has been eaten, the memory is as likely to tantalize our appetite as it is to satisfy us. How much more rewarding would it be if we were able to access a feeling of delight without having to seek it outside ourselves?

Experiencing ecstasy

Here's the good news: ecstasy is within us. Chasing cravings is never going to give us peace, because we're looking in the wrong place. Seeking sensations to slot into our consciousness from outside, as it were, is a distraction from the delights of consciousness itself. In order to feel true ecstasy, we first have to stop, listen, and feel the present moment in all its vibrant, living glory.

Ecstasy is different than pleasure. It's a moment of full participation in ourselves, and in the world – and, if you like to think of it it that way, in the cosmos itself.

Have you ever had a moment when you were out for a walk, watching a beautiful moonrise, dancing to music, where you became so absorbed in what you were doing – the sight, the sounds, the scent and feel of the air on your skin – that the memory stayed with you

for weeks or years afterwards? Even if it lasted only a few seconds, that was an experience of ecstasy. That is what Tantric sex is for: to bring that experience into our love lives, combining the delights of transcendent awareness with the delights of sexuality.

When we say "transcendence," we don't mean rising above our experience. We rise with our experience, partaking of it so fully that it becomes a moment of pure consciousness, relaxing and thrilling at the same time.

Bring your attention to the present moment. You don't have to think or feel the "right" things: when you're truly there, whatever you're experiencing becomes deeply, magically right.

The Meaning of Ecstasy

The word is used a lot in discussing Tantra, but where does it come from? Its origin is the Greek word *ekstasis*, which literally means "outstanding," or a better translation, "standing outside oneself." We don't stop being ourselves when we feel ecstasy, but we stop feeling that we're just ourselves. We become immersed in something outside our regular consciousness, and it is magical.

Understanding

Approachable explanations of the central concepts in Tantric lovemaking are provided to give the reader a good grasp of the basics.

Exercises

The book covers both spiritual and physical exercises you can use to deepen your Tantric experience—some to be tried solo, and some with a partner.

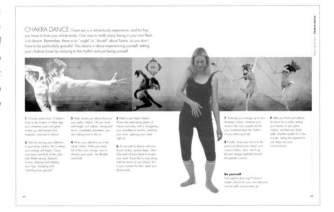

CHAKRA DANCE Great sex is a whole-body experience, and for that, you have to love your whole body. One way to really enjoy being in your own flesh is to dance. Remember, there is no "ought" or "should" about Tantra, so you don't have to be particularly graceful. This dance is about experiencing yourself, setting your chakras loose by swaying to the rhythm and just being yourself.

1 Choose some music. It doesn't have to be Eastern or New Age: pick whatever style and genre makes you feel sexiest and happiest, and start to dance.

2 Start by moving your attention to your base chakra: this is where your energy will begin. Close your eyes and think of the color red. Make strong, dynamic moves, shaking and rotating your hips, stamping and "standing your ground."

3 Next, move your dance focus to your pelvic chakra. Fill your mind with bright, rich yellow. Swing and twist, completely shameless, as you are making love to the air.

4 Move your attention up to the navel chakra. With your mind full of the color orange, start to shimmy your waist – be flexible and bold!

5 Here is your heart chakra. Picture the welcoming green of nature and sway with it, bopping your shoulders to and fro, whirling your arms, opening your chest right up.

6 As you start to dance with your throat chakra, picture deep, clear blue and roll your head to loosen your neck. If you like to sing along with the music as your dance, this is your moment for that: open your throat wide.

7 Drawing your energy up to your third-eye chakra, immerse your mind in the color purple and let your forehead lead the rhythm of your dancing body.

8 Finally, move your focus to the point just above your head, your crown chakra. Spin, reach up: let your energy explode toward the greater cosmos.

9 After you finish your dance, lie down for a while, resting your hands on your pelvic chakra, and feel your body settle. Breathe quietly for a few minutes, letting the experience sink deep into your consciousness.

Be yourself
Not used to dancing? It doesn't matter: dance for your own pleasure and let self-consciousness go.

Step by step

Clear and detailed illustrations will take you through the stages of Tantric rituals and techniques to make it easy, even for beginners, to take their first steps into Tantric pleasures.

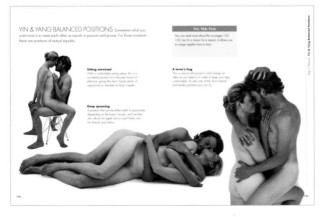

YIN & YANG BALANCED POSITIONS Sometimes what you want most is to meet each other as equals in passion and power. For those moments, these are positions of mutual equality.

Sitting entwined
With a comfortable resting place, this is a wonderful position for a leisurely trance of pleasure, giving the man's hands plenty of opportunity to stimulate his lady's nipples.

Deep spooning
A position that can be either restful or passionate depending on the lovers' moods, and one that also allows his upper arm to roam freely over her breasts and clitoris.

The Tab-Yam

You can read more about this on pages 152–153, but it's a classic for a reason: it allows you to merge together face to face.

A lover's hug
This is one to roll around in and change as often as you need to in order to keep your legs comfortable. It's also one of the most natural and tender positions you can try.

Introduction:
What is Tantric Sex?

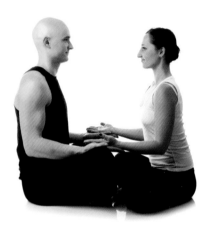

New beginnings

Through Tantric practices, we can free ourselves from old inhibitions and find a new experience of joy.

Tantric sex is one of those phrases that most of us have heard somewhere—but if we get down to specifics, most of us find that, actually, we're not sure what it means. Probably we've heard the stories about how certain celebrities can make love for hours using magical techniques, but what are those techniques? And is making love for hour upon hour actually possible—or even still fun after the first hour or two?

The answer can be yes—but the essence of Tantra is that we broaden our understanding of sexuality. Despite how interested we generally are in sex, and how much time we spend thinking, dreaming, fantasizing, and reading about it, the truth is that we also spend a lot of time worrying about it, or feeling disappointed or inadequate.

Tantra is an ancient set of practices that has been adopted and adapted by every culture it settled in. Its message is about breaking down barriers. Sex and spirit are not two sides of the same coin in this tradition: they are intimately intertwined. We suffer from a lot of such dualities, in fact, and Tantra is there to free us from them. Activity and meditation are opposites? Not necessarily. Peacefulness and excitement can't happen at once? Actually, they can. We're either perfect or imperfect? Not at all: we are both and neither at once. Tantric insight is here to free us from the limiting ideas that stifle our natural capacity for joy.

This process of freedom doesn't just come from insight and meditation,

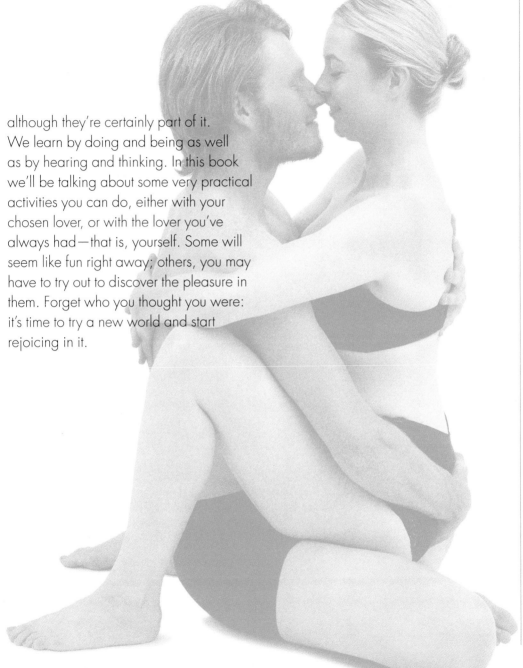

although they're certainly part of it.
We learn by doing and being as well
as by hearing and thinking. In this book
we'll be talking about some very practical
activities you can do, either with your
chosen lover, or with the lover you've
always had—that is, yourself. Some will
seem like fun right away; others, you may
have to try out to discover the pleasure in
them. Forget who you thought you were:
it's time to try a new world and start
rejoicing in it.

Tantric Sex
Worldwide Traditions

The history of Tantra is long, multicultural, and often shrouded in mystery. Its earliest practices seem to have begun in India around the second and third century CE, although some people believe that its roots may go back still further. What we do know is that the Indian practice proved influential throughout Asia, and as Tantra spread across the continent, it adapted to new cultures. Tantra is not a religion—rather it's a kind of religious practice that can be incorporated into any number of faiths, or indeed, non-faiths. Nowadays, you can practice Tantra within the context of a religion if you choose, but it's also possible to approach it as a secular learner.

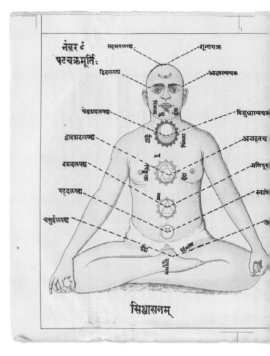

Hinduism

The word "Hinduism" itself refers to a range of different religious groups, and includes many different deities and ideas. The common ground between these religious groups is usually the major scriptures: the *Vedas*, written between 1400 and 400 BCE, the *Upanishads*, written between 800 and 600 BCE, and the *Bhagavad Gita*, probably written at some point between 400 BCE and 200 CE. Hindu doctrines generally rest on the idea that we are born into an endless cycle of reincarnation, and the karma we accrue during our lifetime—that is, the spiritual consequences of our actions and choices—will affect our next rebirth.

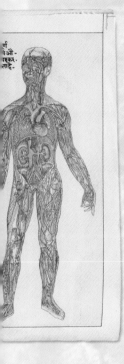

Chakras
The concept of chakras is a long tradition in several Indian religions, and is central to the understanding of Tantric sex.

The aspiration is to finally escape this cycle, through righteous living and enlightenment, and achieve moksha: union with Brahman, the universal soul.

Tantra arrived as a wild and disruptive tradition within Hinduism. It arose from Shaivism—that is, worship of Shiva, one of the three central deities. In Hinduism,

11

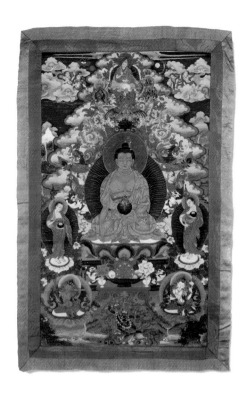

Buddhist roots
Buddhist philosophy remains a strong influence on Tantra to this day.

Brahma is considered the creator god, Vishnu the preserver of the world, and Shiva the god who destroys the universe in order to recreate it. Rather than patiently working our way toward enlightenment through lifetimes of virtue and renunciation, Shaivist Tantra promised a quick route to enlightenment through dramatic experience. The movement certainly wasn't all about sex then (it still isn't nowadays), but it did sweep aside the belief that sex was to be avoided. Instead, it rejected the dualism between spirit and flesh.

Sexuality was energy, energy was divine, and therefore sex could be as good a way to enlightenment as any.

As it has been practiced in Hindu traditions, Tantric rituals involve not just meditation, but also food, dancing, sex, and other physical delights. Followers honor both Shiva and Shakti, his female incarnation and sometimes his consort. Shiva symbolizes consciousness and the eternal masculine, while Shakti symbolizes pure energy, nature, and the eternal feminine. Sex can be one way in which partners embody these two principles—though in modern Tantra, sex doesn't have to involve a man and a woman (see Gender & Love, pages 116–117). Through sexual union, Tantrikas seek to create a union between the principles of the universe that ignites a brilliant spiritual transformation.

Tantra in India reached its height in the eleventh and twelfth centuries CE before declining. During this period it often intertwined with schools of yoga, as both traditions involve transforming the body to transform the spirit—an overlap that continues to this day.

Buddhism

Around 800 CE, Tantra spread as far as Cambodia and other Buddhist nations.

Buddhism was ready to embrace Tantra; Mahayana Buddhism had already been engaged in ritual and magical traditions since the fifth century, making Tantric ideas a natural fit for some religious groups.

In Buddhism, the fundamental belief is that life is a cycle of suffering created by craving and lack of insight, and that, through meditation, we can transcend this cycle and achieve enlightenment or Buddhahood. A great deal of its philosophy focuses on rising above the constraints of dualistic thinking, because seeing ourselves and the cosmos as two opposed entities limits our spiritual insight. Tantra, which sweeps aside the idea that flesh and spirit must be opposites, was a natural fit for Buddhism, and much of contemporary Tantra still rests on this idea.

Taoism

As Tantra spread to China in the early eighth century, it found a new home in Taoist traditions. Taoism, which already had a long history of mutual borrowing of ideas with Buddhism, is perhaps closer to a philosophy than a religion: based on the *Tao Te Ching*, a series of short poetic meditations written in the sixth century by the sage Laozi (or Lao Tzu), Taoism is a path that seeks a healthful balance between all things. Its most familiar icon is probably the yin–yang symbol, the dark and light intertwined with one another and each

Shiva and Shakti

The Hindu deities Shiva and Shakti, representing consciousness and power, embrace in a union both sexual and mystical.

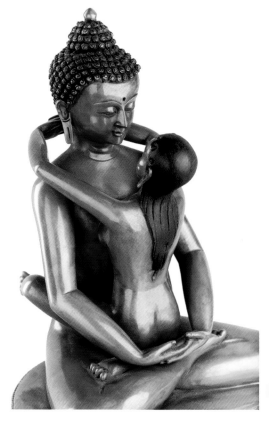

containing a circle of the other at its very center. Yin and yang aren't unique to Taoism, but they are a concept that has long been part of Tantra. (For more discussion, see pages 44–45.)

Contemporary Tantra

Tantra has never been absent from our history since it first developed, but in the twentieth century interest enjoyed an upsurge in the West. This new tradition is sometimes called Neo-Tantra (or, more jokily, "California Tantra," California's various liberated subcultures having been active adopters of the tradition). For the purposes of this book, we will basically be discussing Neo-Tantra, the modern school that takes a great interest in developing our natural life force energy, of which sexuality is one branch.

No kind of Tantra is exclusively about sex, and for some Tantrikas, sex is only a minor aspect. There are plenty of contemporary practitioners of this kind, and you may like to seek out a teacher if you're interested (see some advice about this on page 33), but you don't need to follow that path to enjoy the

sexual delights. This is a book for beginners, and particularly for couples, who are curious about how they can use Tantra to enliven and perhaps even transform their love lives. When so many cultures see sex as dirty and unspiritual, a practice that treats our sexual energy as vital, even sacred, can be a wonderful way of deepening intimacy in our relationships—both with our lovers and with our own bodies, and perhaps even with our own souls.

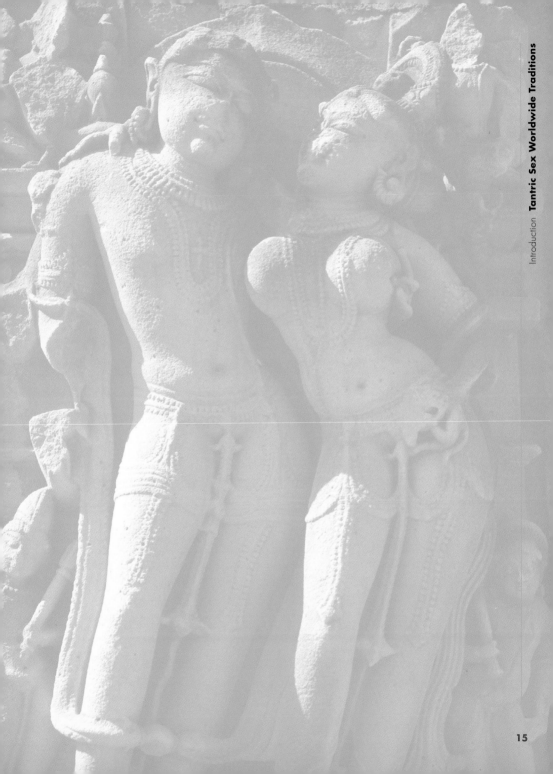

15

PREPARING THE SPIRIT

The natural state for Tantric sex is to be both alert and relaxed. While many of us are used to thinking of mind and body as two separate things, the reality is that, as the saying goes, "the biggest sex organ is the brain." It's our minds that process pleasure, that fantasize and catch light with desire, that create our moods and make us the sexual, joyful creatures that we are. For this reason, the first step on the Tantric path is to become at ease with our minds and our selves. If you have a partner, you may like to meditate together, but it's vital to feel good in ourselves before we can feel good with someone else, so these are mostly solo practices. In this chapter, we'll learn exercises that help us experience the flow of energy and ecstasy that is at the heart of Tantric sex.

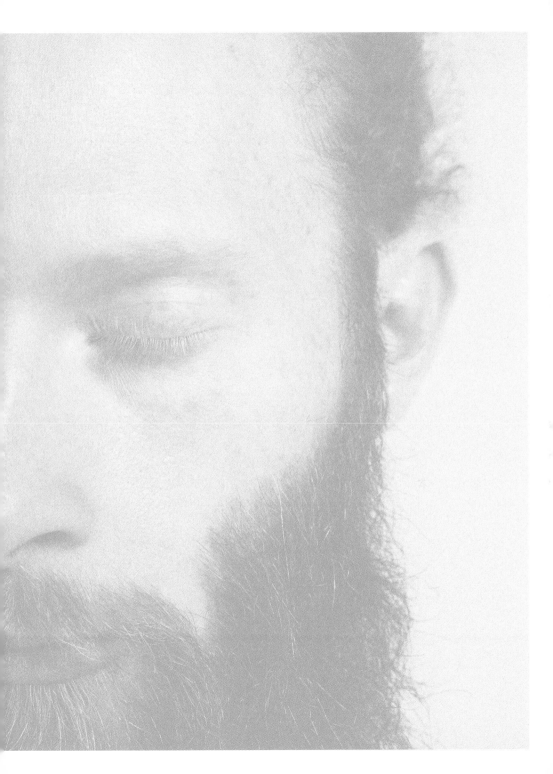

Myths Debunked

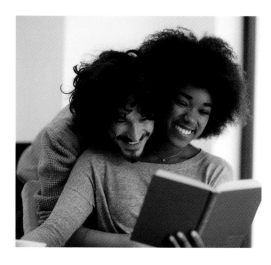

Embrace the experience
*Tantra is far easier to enjoy
than we might fear.*

Sex, like many things we do in private and care about deeply, can be surrounded by half-truths and outright mistakes. Let's begin by sweeping away a few myths so they don't spoil your enjoyment of Tantric lovemaking.

Sex is dirty

Many religions believe there's something immoral about sex—at least, unless it's done in very specific circumstances, probably between a decorous married couple. In Tantra, the body and the soul are a blissful whole, and there is nothing wrong in delighting in them both together. Of course, Tantra isn't an excuse for genuinely unethical behavior—it hurts your spirit as well as others' if you coerce or manipulate someone for sex—but if you honor yourself and your partner, your conscience should be clear.

Sex should go great if you have the right partner

Of course it helps to have someone you find attractive, compatible, and charming, but that doesn't mean you don't get better with practice. Arousal isn't entirely outside our control: on the contrary, we can train our bodies and minds to experience much greater pleasures than we could find if we just let things take their "natural" course.

To enjoy Tantric sex, you have to be a certain type of person

Far from it: Tantra has been practiced in different nations and faiths throughout history, and nowadays it's practiced by people of no particular faith at all. Of course you can go deep into the philosophy if you choose, but the sexual techniques are open to everyone.

Nor do you have to be young or old, straight or gay, New Age or conventional, kinky or vanilla, or anything else. You just have to be you.

Tantra is about penetrative sex going on for hours

You can certainly give it a go if you like, but Tantra is about a much broader approach than that. It's about the flow of energy and being open to divine and earthly pleasures.

Tantra is very difficult to learn

If you're enriching your life, then you're doing Tantric sex. The techniques that we'll study here do repay practice, but remember: any fun, joy, or pleasure you get out of them, no matter what kind, is part of the Tantric process.

Understanding Ecstasy

If you start studying Tantric sex, you'll hear the word "ecstasy" mentioned a lot. It sounds wonderful—but what, in this context, does it actually mean?

Human beings are experience-seekers, and yet experiences can often leave us feeling a little flat. A rollercoaster gives us a rush of adrenaline, and for a short time we're euphoric, but after a while, the feeling settles down and we start to want more. A delicious meal is comforting, but once it has been eaten, the memory is as likely to tantalize our appetite as it is to satisfy us. How much more rewarding would it be if we were able to access a feeling of delight without having to seek it outside ourselves?

Experiencing ecstasy

Here's the good news: ecstasy is within us. Chasing cravings is never going to give us peace, because we're looking in the wrong place. Seeking sensations to slot into our consciousness from outside, as it were, is a distraction from the delights of consciousness itself. In order to feel true ecstasy, we first have to stop, listen, and feel the present moment in all its vibrant, living glory.

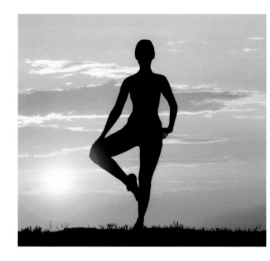

Feel the moment
When we are gladly present in the moment, any experience can become ecstatic.

Ecstasy is different than pleasure. It's a moment of full participation: in ourselves, and in the world—and, if you like to think of it that way, in the cosmos itself.

Have you ever had a moment when you were out for a walk, watching a beautiful moonrise, dancing to music, where you became so absorbed in what you were doing—the sight, the sounds, the scent and feel of the air on your skin—that the memory stayed with you for weeks or years afterward? Even if it lasted only a few seconds, that was an experience of ecstasy. That is what Tantric sex is for: to bring that experience into our love lives, combining the delights of transcendent awareness with the delights of sexuality.

When we say "transcendence," we don't mean rising above our experience. We rise *with* our experience, partaking of it so fully that it becomes a moment of pure consciousness, relaxing and thrilling at the same time.

Bring your attention to the present moment. You don't have to think or feel the "right" things: when you're truly there, whatever you're experiencing becomes deeply, magically right.

The Meaning of Ecstasy

The word is used a lot in discussing Tantra, but where does it come from? Its origin is the Greek word *ekstasis*, which literally means "out-standing," or a better translation, "standing outside oneself." We don't stop being ourselves when we feel ecstasy, but we stop feeling like we're *just* ourselves. We become immersed in something outside our regular consciousness, and it is magical.

Meditation & Insight

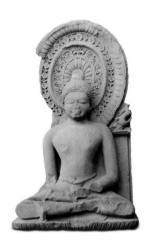

Evidence
According to the archaeological evidence, humans have been meditating since at least 5000 BCE.

Tantric sex depends on enjoying a vibrant, blissful awareness of the present moment. For a modern individual, this doesn't always come naturally: the busy pace of our lives means that we're often adapted to a scurrying mental pace that can be hard to relax. And if we can't relax into blissful awareness, it's not surprising that even if we want sex, when we get to the bedroom we may find it harder to get into things than we could wish. How, then, do we learn to enjoy the delicious present moment? The best way is simply to practice—and that means meditation. An ancient practice, yet advocated today by modern science, it's surprisingly easy to learn, and can enrich your life from the moment you start.

Ancient tradition

In South Asia, spreading through Afghanistan, Pakistan, and Northwest India, lies the Indus Valley, and there is found the first evidence of meditation: sculptures dating back as far as 5000 BCE, sitting cross-legged with their eyes half-closed in a pose of peace and alertness. These artistic representations show us just how deep in human history the practice goes. Since those days, many religions have adopted the process, and in modern life, psychologists and doctors are increasingly recommending meditation to patients for reasons ranging from anxiety to chronic pain. Mystics and scientists alike have come to the simple insight: awareness is good for us.

Meditation techniques

There are many meditation techniques, and we'll describe some simple ones in this chapter, but the principle of all these techniques remains the same: we relax our chattering minds, neither looking back to memories nor thinking ahead to the future, and let ourselves experience life in the present tense.

If that sounds difficult, it is—and it isn't. The human mind is a lively and active organ, and it's almost inevitable that during most meditations, yours will wander. That's to be expected, and the practice allows for it: you simply notice, without judgment, that your mind has strayed from the moment, and return your focus to where it was before.

You may have to do this regularly. Think of it like an endearing animal you're encouraging to sit on a cushion: it will sometimes wander off, because that's what animals do. There's no point blaming it; instead, you just gently scoop it up and put it back, and carry on. Everything is there for you to notice, including the ways your own mind works.

What you are doing is cultivating a state of mindfulness: a gentle consciousness in which you notice all that you are thinking and feeling without any struggle to change it. In this way, you create a space in which ecstasy is free to arise.

BASIC BREATHING MEDITATION

The "mindful breathing" meditation is one of the most ancient and traditional of all, and is recommended by doctors and psychologists as well as Tantric practitioners. It can be done anywhere you have fifteen or twenty minutes to spare. Tantric sex depends on enjoying a vibrant, blissful awareness of the present moment.

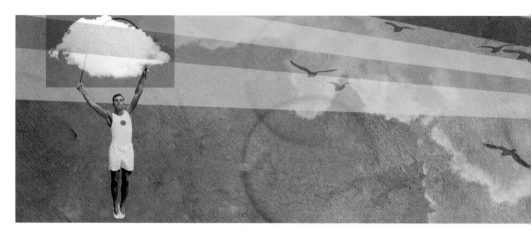

1 *Seat yourself somewhere comfortable. Traditionally this meditation is done cross-legged, but if that's awkward for you, a chair or sofa is fine. Rest your hands on your lap, palms up and relaxed. Close your eyes.*

2 *Gently bring your awareness to your breathing. Feel your stomach or chest rise and fall, the coolness of air in your throat. For about five minutes, focus on the out breath, and count ten exhalations, going back to one again after ten. If you lose count, just go back to one. Let the sensation of breathing out relax you.*

3 *Shift your attention to the in breath. Again, count lightly to ten, feeling your body draw in life-giving oxygen. Experience yourself being filled with energy.*

Mindful breathing
For a breathing meditation, choose a pose that's upright and alert, but doesn't overstrain your body.

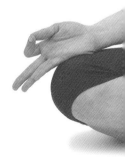

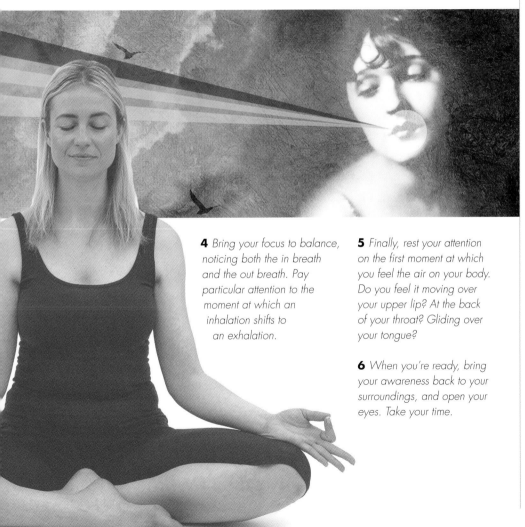

4 Bring your focus to balance, noticing both the in breath and the out breath. Pay particular attention to the moment at which an inhalation shifts to an exhalation.

5 Finally, rest your attention on the first moment at which you feel the air on your body. Do you feel it moving over your upper lip? At the back of your throat? Gliding over your tongue?

6 When you're ready, bring your awareness back to your surroundings, and open your eyes. Take your time.

SENSUAL BREATHING MEDITATION
Having tried a classic mindful breathing meditation, you're now ready for a more sensual breathing meditation. This is a self-pleasuring exercise: your first lover is always yourself, and you can only become a better lover of others by enjoying your own body.

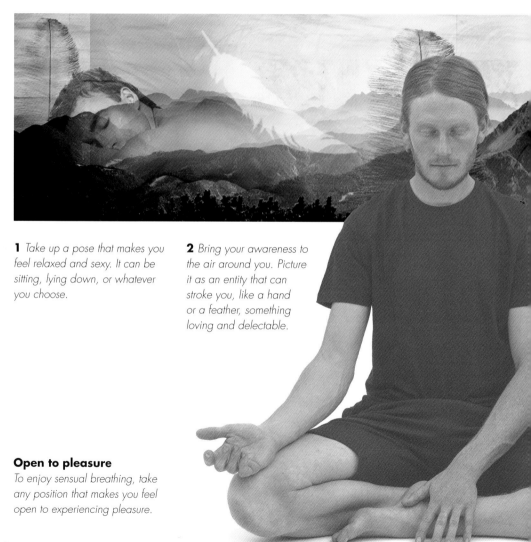

1 Take up a pose that makes you feel relaxed and sexy. It can be sitting, lying down, or whatever you choose.

2 Bring your awareness to the air around you. Picture it as an entity that can stroke you, like a hand or a feather, something loving and delectable.

Open to pleasure
To enjoy sensual breathing, take any position that makes you feel open to experiencing pleasure.

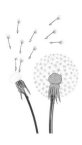

Relax and drift

*Let your awareness drift into
a state of soft, tranquil arousal.*

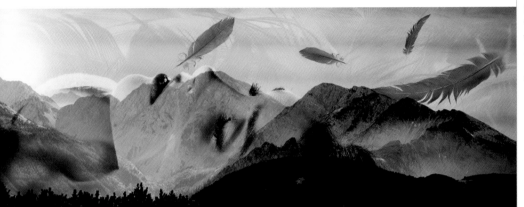

3 *As you draw in your breath, feel how the air moves around and inside you. Relax into the sensation, letting the world pleasure you.*

4 *As you exhale, experience how your breath is going out into the caressing world. Picture it as if you are responding to the air's touch by sending out your energy to reciprocate its tenderness.*

5 *Let your sensual awareness spread throughout your body. With each breath, draw the energy down as deep as you can, until you feel an echo in your genitals.*

6 *Carry on as long as the exercise is enjoyable.*

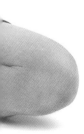

LOVING-KINDNESS MEDITATION

Sex isn't just a matter of physical sensation; it's also a matter of emotion. We think and worry a great deal about romantic love, but there's a traditional Buddhist meditation that can help you feel love in a wider context. Known in Pali as the "metta bhavana," meaning the

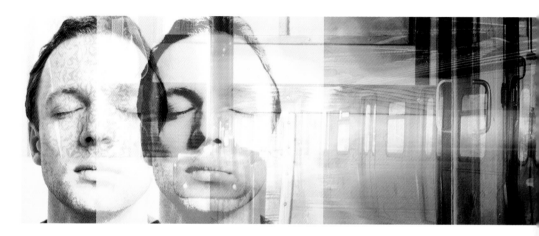

1 *Sitting comfortably, cultivate a feeling of loving-kindness, and direct it toward yourself. Wish yourself well, and appreciate yourself as the precious being you are. You may like to repeat a phrase such as "May I be well and happy" or picture a warm, golden light embracing you.*

2 *Now think of a person you're fond of—preferably not a lover, parent, or child, as such feelings are often complicated and bound up with our own needs, but someone you find it easy to wish well. Picture that person, and focus a feeling of loving-kindness on them.*

3 *Think of a stranger, somebody you know only slightly, such as a clerk at your local store or a fellow commuter you sometimes see on the train. Send them loving kindness, and sincerely wish them safe and joyous.*

Cultivate kindness
Take a little time to cultivate kindness: it'll warm your whole body and spirit.

cultivation of loving-kindness, it's a wonderful meditation to ground yourself in a positive attitude. Even if the sex you prefer to have is casual rather than romantic, loving-kindness is a fine foundation: it helps you view others warmly, and gives you a deep sense of emotional security from which to take flight.

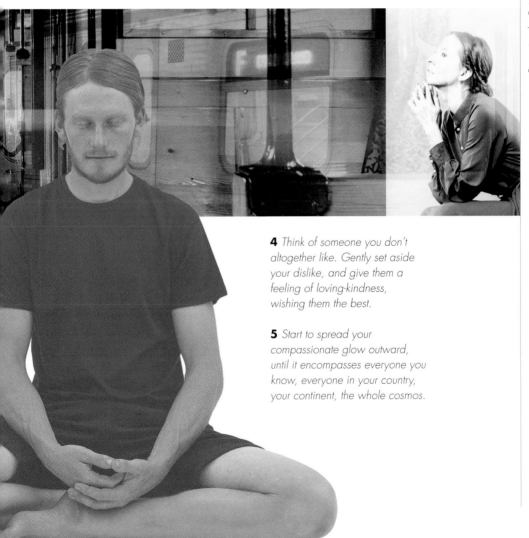

4 *Think of someone you don't altogether like. Gently set aside your dislike, and give them a feeling of loving-kindness, wishing them the best.*

5 *Start to spread your compassionate glow outward, until it encompasses everyone you know, everyone in your country, your continent, the whole cosmos.*

THE INNER SMILE MEDITATION

It's a traditional Taoist belief that we can benefit both our bodies and our spirits by sending a daily smile to our inner organs. Part of the system of Neidan, or Inner Alchemy, this is a lovely way to develop a positive attitude toward the miraculous creation that is your body.

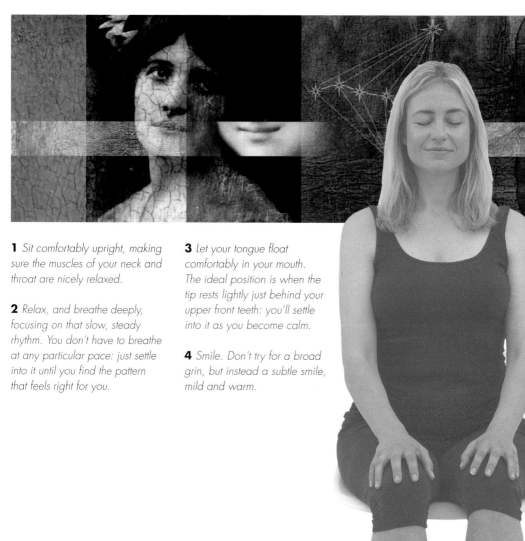

1 *Sit comfortably upright, making sure the muscles of your neck and throat are nicely relaxed.*

2 *Relax, and breathe deeply, focusing on that slow, steady rhythm. You don't have to breathe at any particular pace: just settle into it until you find the pattern that feels right for you.*

3 *Let your tongue float comfortably in your mouth. The ideal position is when the tip rests lightly just behind your upper front teeth: you'll settle into it as you become calm.*

4 *Smile. Don't try for a broad grin, but instead a subtle smile, mild and warm.*

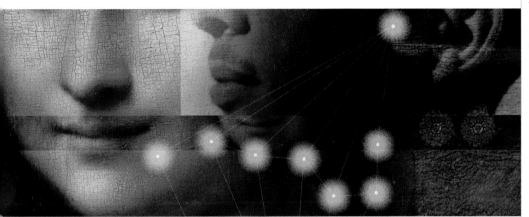

5 *Bring your attention to your third-eye chakra. Your energy will start to gather there, and as it does, draw it back to the space Taoists call the Crystal Palace: the center of your brain, right between your ears.*

6 *Send this energy back to your eyes, letting them develop the smile. Imagine them developing a tender and loving gaze.*

7 *In your imagination, direct that gaze toward whatever part of your body most needs love—perhaps your genitals, or a part of you that you fear is unattractive. Give it the inner smile energy until it feels energized and safe.*

8 *When you're satisfied, finally draw your energy down into your navel chakra, letting the smile spread through you. Release your tongue, and smile openly until you feel ready to stop.*

Smiling eyes
When you develop "smiling eyes," you have the power to create a healing inner gaze.

31

Honoring the Self

We all want to be loved, and many of us would like to have a lover who excites our senses and cares for our well-being. Tantra can turn a good relationship into a great one, but there's something else to remember: we have to love ourselves.

Self-love

Self-love in all its forms can be an uncomfortable subject. We have plenty of words for people who seem to love themselves too much—vain, arrogant, stuck-up, selfish. What's important to understand, though, is that a glad appreciation of who you are is not a bad thing. It is, on the contrary, the foundation of the ability to love at all. It's hard to love anyone or anything healthily when there's a hole in our heart that needs to be filled. When we're confident in ourselves, it's far easier to appreciate others.

Self-pleasuring

The same can be said of "self-love" in the sense of masturbation—or, to put it more attractively, self-pleasuring. From rough jokes to religious prohibitions, it is

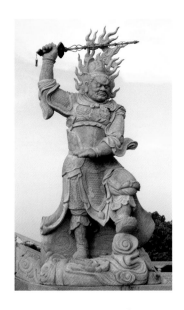

Inner strength
Being spiritual does not mean being weak or self-destructive. Use your power to protect your well-being.

frequently a taboo subject. It's time to let those ideas go. Pleasuring ourselves is as natural and simple an act as drinking when we're thirsty or stretching when we've been sitting for too long. A good relationship with your own sensations is the foundation of a happy sex life.

A final word on honoring the self: honoring something includes protecting it from harm. Choose your lovers carefully, and don't stay with someone who doesn't treat you kindly. Insist on whatever safe sex precautions you deem necessary, and feel free to reject any lover who doesn't respect them. If you're interested in finding a teacher to learn more about Tantric ideas, remember that every appealing philosophy attracts some unscrupulous characters, so don't be afraid to "vet" potential gurus and avoid any who seem manipulative. Tantra does involve transcendence, but that doesn't mean it's unspiritual to pay attention to your own doubts if a lover or teacher seems to be doing something unreasonable. You are your own best protector: cherish yourself as you would any other precious thing.

LETTING GO

Are you holding on to any old shames, disappointments, insecurities, or frustrations? It's time to take their burden off your spirit and put it in the past, where it belongs. In this exercise you write your old experiences, let them flow out of your hand, onto the page, and away.

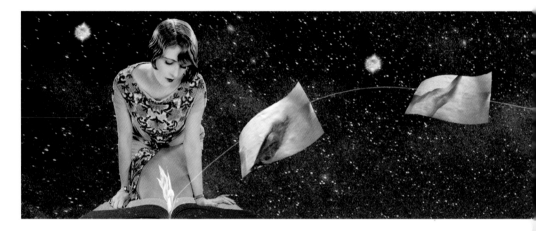

1 *Get yourself ready with some loose sheets of paper and a pen. The paper needn't be fancy; in fact, it's probably better if it's cheap. Relax yourself with a mindful breathing meditation (see pages 24–25).*

2 *Think through your past history. What are the times when you felt ashamed for being too sexual? For instance, were you embarrassed over a crush? Told that "good girls" or "good boys" don't touch themselves? Rejected unkindly when you tried to seduce a partner? Write it down.*

3 *Were there times when you felt you might not be sexual enough? For instance, were you a "late bloomer"? Did you have a partner who wanted sex more than you did? Have you had times of feeling undesirable? Write those memories down too.*

Lighten the spirit

Writing down past issues won't make you forget them, but it can lessen the power they have over you.

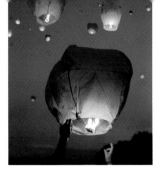

Release the burden

Let your past dissatisfactions float away and clear a path for new experiences.

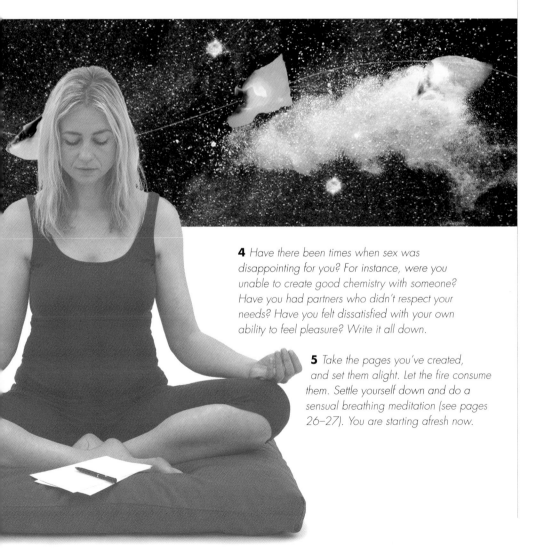

4 *Have there been times when sex was disappointing for you? For instance, were you unable to create good chemistry with someone? Have you had partners who didn't respect your needs? Have you felt dissatisfied with your own ability to feel pleasure? Write it all down.*

5 *Take the pages you've created, and set them alight. Let the fire consume them. Settle yourself down and do a sensual breathing meditation (see pages 26–27). You are starting afresh now.*

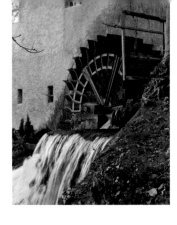

Energy flow
When nothing is blocking us, our energy can flow with all its natural power.

CHAKRAS

What exactly is a chakra? The word comes from the Sanskrit, and literally means "wheel." In yogic tradition, we are thought to have seven chakras, each corresponding to a set of organs within our bodies, each with its own particular function and associated with a set of emotions.

It's helpful to think of the seven chakras as a series of water-wheels or pipes. Energy flows through each of them—but if one of the chakras becomes blocked, then energy can't move through it freely, and our bodies and spirits stop working as they should do.

Clean flow

A great deal of Tantric sex depends on letting energy flow cleanly through your body, so as you consider your chakras, consider whether any insecurities, frustrations, or sorrows may be creating obstacles for you. If so, don't panic: life is a dynamic process and your emotions are far more fluid than they seem. Treat yourself with kindness and act as honorably as you can, and your chakras should start to come free again.

Understanding

Chakras are an ancient concept, and modern practitioners differ on how literally they take the idea. For Tantric sex, they are a useful way of thinking about how we relate to ourselves: whether you believe they are physical phenomena or just helpful metaphors, it's crucial to understand chakras in order to understand how Tantric sex is conceived. Whatever interpretation makes sense to you, go with it: exploring your chakras is the pathway into Tantric pleasures.

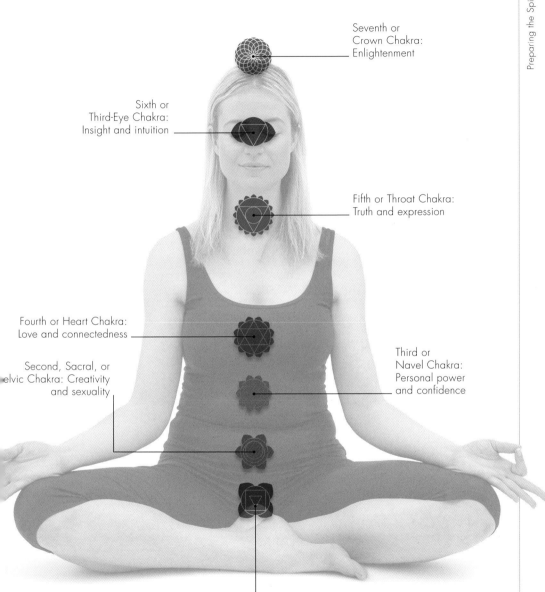

Seventh or
Crown Chakra:
Enlightenment

Sixth or
Third-Eye Chakra:
Insight and intuition

Fifth or Throat Chakra:
Truth and expression

Fourth or Heart Chakra:
Love and connectedness

Third or
Navel Chakra:
Personal power
and confidence

Second, Sacral, or
Pelvic Chakra: Creativity
and sexuality

First or Root Chakra:
Survival, security, and belonging

The First Chakra

Other names:
Root Chakra, *Muladhara*

Color: Red

Element: Earth

Parts of the body:
Base of spine, colon, and anus

Blocked by: Danger and upheaval

Aspects: The first chakra is associated with grounding, survival, and our most basic needs. On an interpersonal level, this means our community and family: it flows well when we have a sense of safety and belonging. When this chakra is open, we feel strong, fearless, able to "stand on our own two feet."

 ## The Second Chakra

Other names:
Sacral Chakra, Pelvic Chakra, *Svadhisthana*

Color: Orange

Element: Water

Parts of the body:
Pelvis and sexual organs

Blocked by: Violation, trampled boundaries, excessive criticism, shame

Aspects: This is the sexual chakra. More broadly, it's associated with creativity: it's where our organs of generation reside, and imaginatively, it's where our flow of ideas also gains power. When this chakra is open, we are pleasurable, inventive, flexible, and positive.

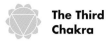 ## The Third Chakra

Other names:
Navel Chakra, Lustrous Gem, *Manipura*

Color: Yellow

Element: Fire

Parts of the body:
Navel to breastbone, digestive organs, and adrenal glands

Blocked by: Fear, anger

Aspects: This is where our "gut feelings" reside: the Navel Chakra is a place of intuition, courage, and self-esteem. When open, it's a place of power—not to hurt others, but to trust and connect with them.

 ## The Fourth Chakra

Other names:
Heart Chakra, *Anahata*

Color: Green

Element: Air

Parts of the body:
Heart, lungs, and arms

Blocked by: Grief, guilt, and bitterness

Aspects: This chakra is a bridge: residing between the lower, more physical chakra and the upper, "spirit" chakras, it is the wheel that turns between body and soul. This is a chakra of balance and unconditional love: we become compassionate toward both ourselves and others, and able to reach out and make healthy connections.

 ## The Fifth Chakra

Other names:
Throat Chakra, *Vishuddha*

Color: Blue

Element: Ether

Parts of the body:
Throat and mouth

Blocked by: Dishonesty and conflict—both with others and within ourselves

Aspects: This is the communication chakra, the part of us that sings out our truth. Sitting between the head and the heart, this is the place where we make our decisions: we can choose to stifle ourselves, or else we can speak honestly, kindly, and as we truly are.

 ## The Sixth Chakra

Other names:
Third-Eye Chakra, *Ajna*

Color: Purple

Element: Light

Parts of the body:
Brain and eyes

Blocked by: Closed-mindedness, logic at the expense of feeling, mistrust

Aspects: Through this chakra we access "vision"—our highest intuitions and insights that see clearly. When we're out of balance, this chakra can try to dominate our instincts, "reasoning" us into positions we don't really believe. Unblocked, it's the site of true clarity and wisdom, perceptive both inside and out.

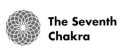

The Seventh Chakra

Other names:
Crown Chakra, Thousand-Petaled Lotus, Sahasrara

Color: White or violet

Element: Cosmic energy

Parts of the body:
Brain, or the space just above the head

Blocked by: Disconnection, spiritual imbalance

Aspects: Through this chakra, we connect to the whole universe. We don't necessarily have an "out of body" experience, but we reach up in surrender and bliss, losing ourselves in something great and benevolent that nourishes and embraces us as part of a blissful whole.

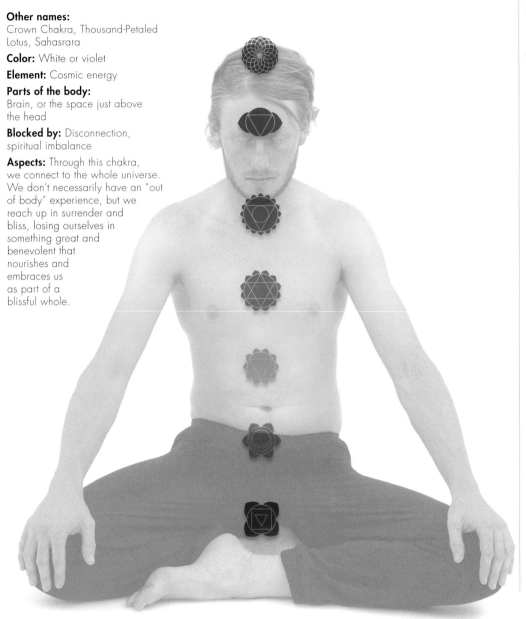

BELLY MEDITATION

How much do you love your stomach? Considering how many "perfect" images we're surrounded by, the answer is very probably "not much at all." Male or female, our tummies are supposed to be tight and flat—despite the fact that it's natural for the body to deposit a little fat there for protection. (Or even plenty of fat. It's all right: it's all you.) As a result, many of us hold our stomachs in.

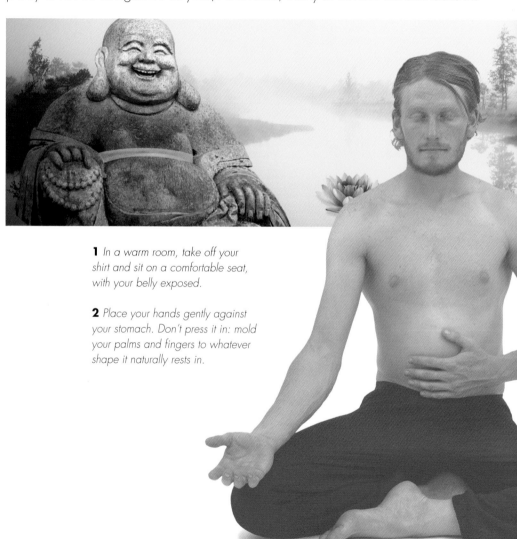

1 *In a warm room, take off your shirt and sit on a comfortable seat, with your belly exposed.*

2 *Place your hands gently against your stomach. Don't press it in: mold your palms and fingers to whatever shape it naturally rests in.*

The stomach, though, contains the chakra most associated with sexual energy (see pages 36–39 for more on chakras): few things will constrain it more than hating the body part that contains it. Who can enjoy free-flowing sexual energy when we can't relax about our middles? It's time to let go of our self-consciousness and enjoy our bellies for the glorious wells of life they are.

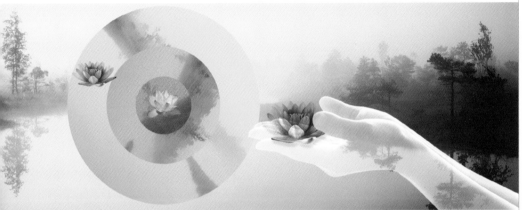

3 *Breathe in deep until your stomach is fully extended. Let it be as big as possible. Smile, and send it warm, positive energy from your hands.*

4 *Release the breath, blowing out any negative feelings. Keep doing this until you feel satisfied. As you perform the belly meditation, let a kind smile rest on your lips, to encourage a warm and happy mood.*

Center of gravity
The stomach is our center of gravity. In loving our belly, we're loving our own stability.

CHAKRA DANCE

Great sex is a whole-body experience, and for that, you have to love your whole body. One way to really enjoy being in your own flesh is to dance. Remember, there is no "ought" or "should" about Tantra, so you don't have to be particularly graceful. This dance is about experiencing yourself, setting your chakras loose by swaying to the rhythm and just being yourself.

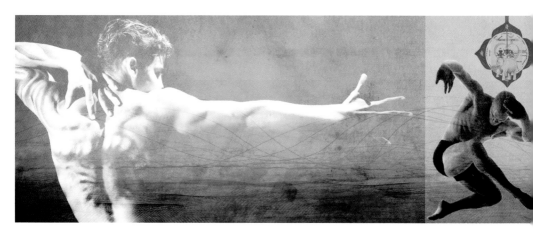

1 *Choose some music. It doesn't have to be Eastern or New Age: pick whatever style and genre makes you feel sexiest and happiest, and start to dance.*

2 *Start by moving your attention to your base chakra: this is where your energy will begin. Close your eyes and think of the color red. Make strong, dynamic moves, shaking and rotating your hips, stamping and "standing your ground."*

3 *Next, move your dance focus to your pelvic chakra. Fill your mind with bright, rich yellow. Swing and thrust, completely shameless: you are making love to the air.*

4 *Move your attention up to the navel chakra. With your mind full of the color orange, start to shimmy your waist—be flexible and bold.*

5 *Next is your heart chakra. Picture the welcoming green of nature and sway with it, boogieing your shoulders to and fro, whirling your arms, opening your chest right up.*

6 *As you start to dance with your throat chakra, picture deep, clean blue and roll your head to loosen your neck. If you like to sing along with the music as you dance, this is your moment for that: open your throat wide.*

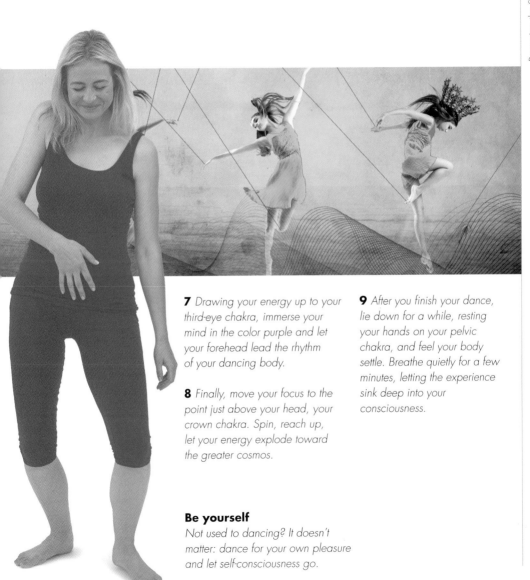

7 *Drawing your energy up to your third-eye chakra, immerse your mind in the color purple and let your forehead lead the rhythm of your dancing body.*

8 *Finally, move your focus to the point just above your head, your crown chakra. Spin, reach up, let your energy explode toward the greater cosmos.*

9 *After you finish your dance, lie down for a while, resting your hands on your pelvic chakra, and feel your body settle. Breathe quietly for a few minutes, letting the experience sink deep into your consciousness.*

Be yourself

Not used to dancing? It doesn't matter: dance for your own pleasure and let self-consciousness go.

Yin & Yang

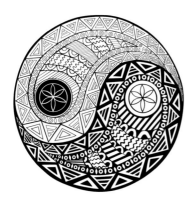

Natural balance

Yin and yang exist in constant interplay, and each, at its heart, contains a little of the other.

In Taoist Tantra, and indeed Taoism in general, a central concept is the idea of yin and yang: the idea dates back through Chinese philosophy to as early as the third century BCE. It's a crucial concept for understanding both our own natures, and the nature of the world.

Creation myth

According to one Chinese creation myth, the world was created from a cosmic egg, in which slept the giant Pangu. Yin and yang were in the egg with him, coming into balance, and when Pangu awoke, he split the egg, separating yin and yang. The upper half of the egg became the sky, the lower half became the earth, and eventually he died and his body became the rest of the world.

Balance is central to Taoism, and the yin and yang icon is the illustration of how its sages see the cosmos: an inextricably entwined back-and-forth between opposites, each of which could not exist without the other.

Masculine and feminine

It's important for a modern person to understand that the "masculine" and "feminine" elements don't mean that a male lover must always take the active role and a female lover the passive, or indeed that you need to have both a male and a female lover at play. Gender can be a fluid thing, and contemporary Tantra embraces that (see Gender & Love, pages 116–117). Rather, yin and yang are states that every person contains and can embody. Sometimes you may wish to make love in a state of yang, active and dominant, while sometimes you may prefer to make love in yin, receptive and yielding. There are no rules: you can access both to enrich your lovemaking.

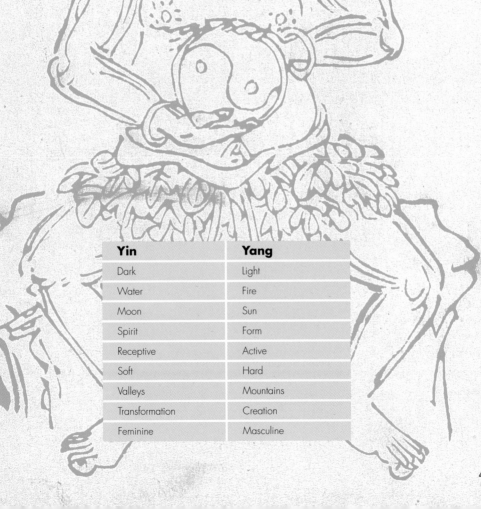

Yin	Yang
Dark	Light
Water	Fire
Moon	Sun
Spirit	Form
Receptive	Active
Soft	Hard
Valleys	Mountains
Transformation	Creation
Feminine	Masculine

THIRD-EYE MEDITATION

In Tantric lovemaking, your body is filled with light. A wonderful way to open yourself up to this is to do a meditation on your upper two chakras—the third-eye chakra, representing insight, and your crown chakra, representing cosmic energy and liberation (see Chakras, pages 36–39).

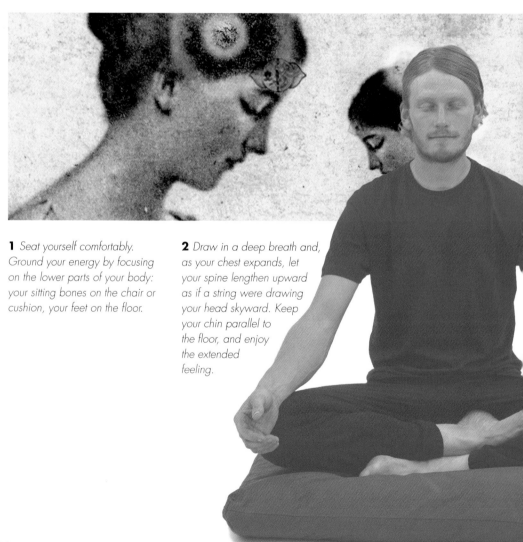

1 *Seat yourself comfortably. Ground your energy by focusing on the lower parts of your body: your sitting bones on the chair or cushion, your feet on the floor.*

2 *Draw in a deep breath and, as your chest expands, let your spine lengthen upward as if a string were drawing your head skyward. Keep your chin parallel to the floor, and enjoy the extended feeling.*

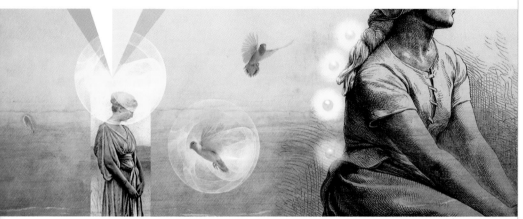

3 *Exhale, and let your tailbone extend downward, connecting you to the earth. Your spine is releasing in both directions.*

4 *Let your tongue float in your mouth as in the Inner Smile meditation (see page 30), and imagine, just in front of your third-eye chakra, a ball of golden light floating in the air. As you inhale through your nose, roll the ball*

over the top of your head, passing along your crown chakra, and then down your spine all the way to your tailbone.

5 *Exhale through your nose, and as you do, roll the ball back up, over your crown chakra and back to your third-eye chakra. Keep rolling the ball back and forth until you're thoroughly energized.*

Posture

Many of us work jobs that aren't great for the posture. By extending our spines, we can lighten the whole body.

The Dream Journal

Do you know what you truly desire? One of the beauties of Tantra is that it helps us to gain intuitive insight; as you open up your mind, you may find longings or curiosities floating to the surface that you didn't know were there. When we sleep, our conscious mind hands over control: the subconscious is in charge, and it whispers to us of what we want. You contain limitless potential, so as you start to release the sexual energy in your spirit, listen to every aspect of yourself. Here's one way to keep a dream journal to accompany you on your journey.

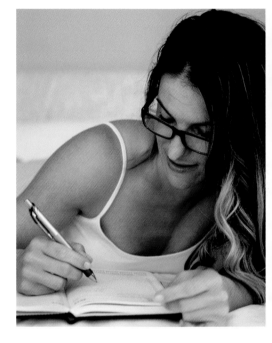

Subconscious messages
Learn to interpret the secret whispers of your subconscious mind.

Choose a book and pen

It may seem like you need a special volume to write in, but actually, you may do better with something fairly ordinary-looking. The reason? Your subconscious and your sexuality aren't something separate and removed from your "normal" experience. If you make the book too fancy, you may feel uncomfortable writing honestly about mundane-seeming dreams, and that will inhibit your truthfulness. The priorities are a book that's easy to write on—hardback covers can help—and a pen that's reliable and feels good to use.

Create a usable space

You don't want to be knocking over your water glass or groping for a pen when you try to write, so set it up to be easy to start writing in a sleepy state.

As you drift off to sleep, do some sensual breathing

(See Sensual Breathing Meditation, pages 26–27.) Your subconscious can't be forced, but it can be enticed. Enjoy the smoothness of your pillow, the warmth of your covers, the weight of your body in the bed, and let sleep embrace you.

When you wake, jot down the key points first

Don't worry about being coherent; dreams usually aren't. Write down vivid images, key words, and strongest emotions. Once you've written those, add more details if you remember them, and see what your dreams might be telling you.

Drawing Up Energy

Having practiced these techniques, you're ready to understand a central concept in Tantric sex: the practice of drawing up energy.

It may sound esoteric, but in fact it's quite simple. For instance, while doing a breathing meditation, did you feel the sensations of your body becoming more intense according to where you placed your attention? You were drawing energy from one place to another. In the Inner Smile meditation (see pages 30–31), did you feel the place you "smiled" at grow warmer, lighter, or heavier? Again, you were sending energy there.

Energy exercise

Try a simple exercise: lie on your bed naked, and hover your hand just above your skin, starting level with your base chakra. Move your hand slowly upward, going from chakra to chakra. Do you feel the warmth of your hand against your skin? You're feeling energy passing from hand to chakra and back. That's what life is: energy within the body, the tangible vibration that keeps us warm, vital—and sexual. As you practice, be aware of how energy is circulating through your body: it makes everything about sex more delightful.

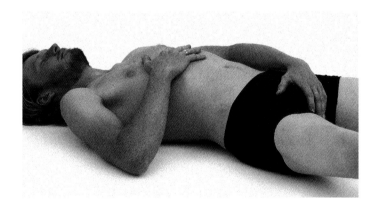

Feel the energy
*Drawing energy from one part of
your body to another can take practice,
but it's delicious practice to do.*

Understanding Energy

In Tantric sex, sexual energy isn't separate
from any other kind of energy: they're all
part of the same dynamic flow. It's this
understanding of energy that is at the center
of Tantric sex. There's nothing about us that
isn't sexual, because "sexual" is simply one
way of describing to ourselves the energy
that rings within our own bodies and within
the cosmos itself.

PREPARING THE BODY

Sex is a physical activity as well as a spiritual one, and in this chapter we will be including some physical exercises. It's important to say, though, that they aren't here to make you thinner, more muscular, or otherwise more like an airbrushed centerfold. Tantric sex is about the flow of energy, and if your body has at least a certain amount of fitness, your energy can flow more freely and for longer. The poses chosen for this chapter will stretch and strengthen the muscles you use in lovemaking, meaning that you'll feel more comfortable, and better able to focus your energy on the delectable sensations you're experiencing. Besides this, it's good to enjoy your body. In this chapter, you'll try both self-acceptance and some light, pleasant physical challenges. Hopefully, as you practice, you'll feel increasingly comfortable in your skin and ready to deepen your physical joy.

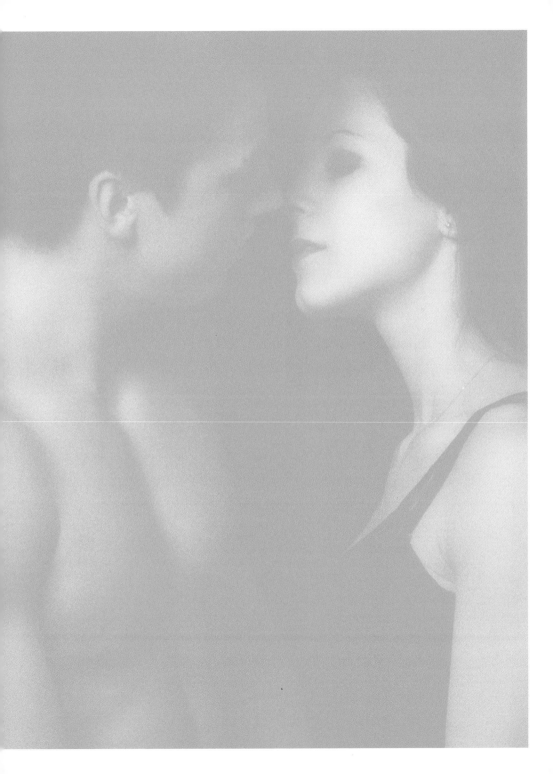

The Meaning of Orgasm

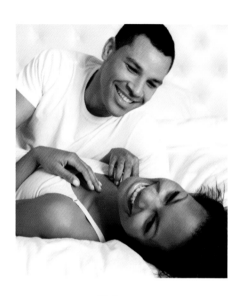

Release

*The true orgasm is a moment of
passionate release, which can
take a wealth of different forms.*

If there's one thing people have heard
about Tantric sex, it's usually that it
makes us capable of having orgasmic
sex for hours at a time. But what exactly
do we mean by an orgasm?

The usual definition is that orgasm is
a sexual climax, a series of muscle
contractions in the genitals that gives us
a feeling of intense pleasure for a few
seconds—around 18 for women and 22
for men, according to current sex research.

Energy climaxes

The first thing to understand is that in
Tantra, the understanding of an orgasm
goes beyond that of a muscular spasm.
Orgasm is a build-up of energy, followed
by a climactic release—and that energy
can take many forms. For instance, have
you ever found yourself laughing so hard
that your energy seems to build to a kind
of "laughtergasm," leaving you exhausted
and relaxed afterward? Or have you ever
felt so passionately that your feelings
have built to an immense crescendo—
something that modern Tantrikas sometimes
call an "emotiongasm"? In Tantra, energy
climaxes are all part of the journey—even
supposedly "negative" feelings such as
anger, fear, or weeping can create that
deep-felt build-and-release.

Deep and total experience

Of course, we all love the sensation of
the genital orgasm, and hopefully as you
follow the Tantric path there will be plenty
of those. The key is not to disregard
the traditional orgasm, but rather to
understand it as part of the broader
picture. A Tantric climax can be any
moment of deep and total experience

that completely overwhelms you and makes you, in that passionate flow of energy, absolutely alive.

Since the ancient days of Tantra, more and more people have been discovering this truth: for instance, the psychoanalyst and sexual freedom activist Wilhelm Reich described orgasm as "the capacity to surrender to the flow of biological energy, free of any inhibition." It is an insight that opens you up to a deeper world of feeling and satisfaction. As you enjoy lovemaking, either with a partner or pleasuring yourself, remain open to the rich range of climaxes you can feel.

Divine Body Acceptance

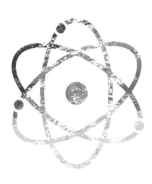

Energy dance

In every atom, particles whirl around each other in a dance of energy. That's what we're made of, and in Tantra, all energy can be sexual energy. We are, in our physical selves, extraordinary.

Most of us have an uncomfortable feeling that our bodies are not as "perfect" as they should be. In Tantric sex, that's just a misconception.

A Tantric lesson: we aren't separate from the universe. We have an individual consciousness, and that consciousness makes us *feel* separate—but this is one of the great misconceptions of the human condition. Think about it: every conscious creature in the world has its own mind and awareness, but does that mean it's not part of the world? Of course not: the world is made up of living things. And if it's not true of them, it isn't true of you, or of any other person. There are limits to how much we're able to perceive and understand our unity with the world, but those are limits—and divine consciousness helps us transcend them.

Sexual energy

The same is true of energy. In Tantra, it is understood that the cosmos is full of sexual energy, because sexual energy isn't separate from the great vibration of the whole universe. Modern physicists will tell you that there's energy in every atom, and that's true of human beings too: we are atoms and matter, thrumming with force and vitality.

And that being the case, anyone who tells you that you aren't "sexy" if you don't fit a certain dress size or can't bench press a certain amount is simply talking nonsense. To be alive is to be sexy; to inhabit a physical body is to be filled with sexual energy.

A sexy lover is someone who makes us feel good. A sexy self is a self capable of feeling good, and of giving pleasure to another. That's just all there is to it. We are, in Tantric sex, embodiments of the great energy of life that echoes through the cosmos—and if we bulge or sag a bit here and there, it just doesn't matter. The face of the sea is wrinkled with waves; the surface of a planet is lumpy and bumpy. We are what we are, and what we are is beautiful.

SELF-ACCEPTANCE EXERCISE

Do you feel good about the way you look? We are each of us a living part of the great universe. There is nothing about us that is not beautiful. This is an exercise that you can do every morning to help you appreciate yourself.

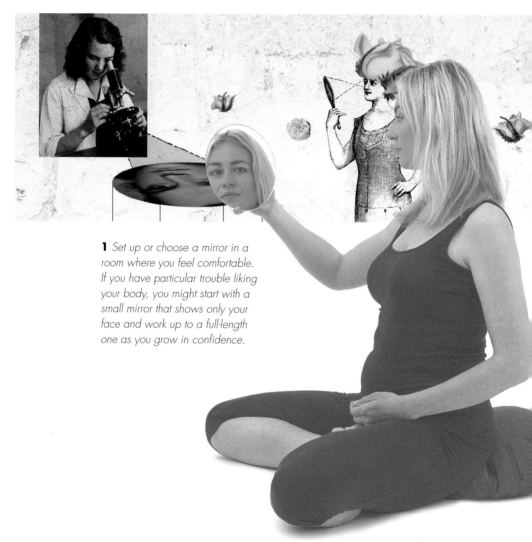

1 *Set up or choose a mirror in a room where you feel comfortable. If you have particular trouble liking your body, you might start with a small mirror that shows only your face and work up to a full-length one as you grow in confidence.*

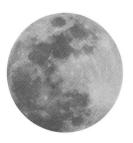

Nobody's perfect

Nothing splendid in the universe is smooth and perfect. Why should we demand it of ourselves?

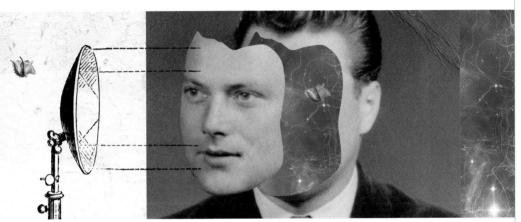

2 *Close your eyes and sit or stand before this mirror. Breathe calmly and deeply, and send some Inner Smile energy (see page 30) to your body, especially the parts of it that you worry about most.*

3 *Repeat to yourself some affirmations. You can use whatever phrases feel best to you; some good starters are:*
- *My body is the vessel of my soul and sexuality.*
- *As the universe is beautiful, I am beautiful.*
- *My body is right, through and through.*

4 *When you feel ready, open your eyes and look at yourself in the mirror. Meet your own gaze kindly.*

5 *Say to yourself, out loud, "[My name], I love you exactly the way you are." Repeat this ten times. If it feels strange, or difficult to say, don't worry: you can feel however you feel. Just keep saying the words.*

6 *Close your eyes and again repeat some affirmations. Rest for a while until you feel calm and ready to face the day.*

You are beautiful

Look at yourself in the same way as you would look at a person you honored and adored.

Kundalini Energy

Kundalini energy is conceived of as a serpent, tucked up at the base of your spine and, when unleashed through activating your chakras, ready to awaken. Contained within that serpent is all the power of your body and spirit.

If you look even briefly into Tantra or yoga, you'll hear the phrase "Kundalini energy." The word comes from Sanskrit and means "coiled," invoking the curled snake that usually represents it.

Feminine power

The Indian tradition conceives of Kundalini as feminine, the Shakti power that travels up the spine to unite with Shiva, her divine consort, at the seventh chakra. (See pages 10–13 for more on Hindu Tantra.) We are releasing the mighty power that drives human development and enlightenment.

A gentle warning: the release of this energy can be very intense, and can, if it comes on too suddenly, leave us feeling disorientated, hypersensitive to stimuli, or struggling to manage our moods and perceptions—a condition called "Kundalini syndrome." If this happens, don't panic: the key is to exercise good self-care: rest, sleep, eat wholesome food, spend time in nature, and give yourself as much peace as you can. If these don't help, seek out a doctor to make sure you're all right. Don't push yourself, and lay off practicing further yoga and meditation until you feel relaxed again.

Spiritual force

Kundalini, then, is energy that can have great power—for blissful experiences as well as for alarming ones. It's for this reason that yoga, which has long been intertwined with Tantric practices, is a spiritual tradition as well as a physical exercise. By unlocking our body's spiritual force, beginning with the root chakra (see pages 36–39 for more on chakras), we access Kundalini energy.

Do as many of these exercises with a partner as you can. Be supportive with each other: there are few better ways to increase your bond and trust than by sharing your experiences. Remember, don't compete or compare—you are not trying to reach a fixed goal, but to open yourselves to whatever comes. Accept the gift of your partner's trust and treat it with the reverence it deserves.

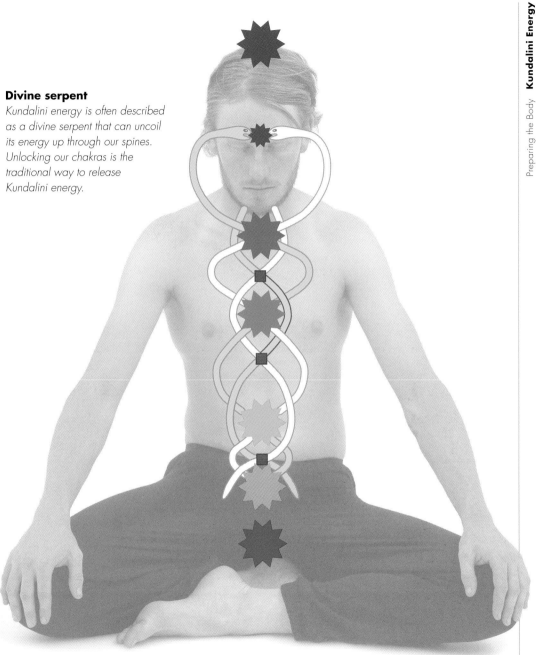

Divine serpent

Kundalini energy is often described as a divine serpent that can uncoil its energy up through our spines. Unlocking our chakras is the traditional way to release Kundalini energy.

Yogic Breathing & the Power of "Edging"

I f you're familiar with modern sexual fads, you may have heard people singing the praises of a practice known as "edging." More formally known as "orgasm control," it's a practice that has been known to Tantric lovers for centuries—in fact, it's central to the Tantric experience.

Teasing

How do we do it? Put simply, the technique means teasing ourselves along the edge of orgasm without ever quite tipping over. It's a technique we can practice either with partners or by ourselves—it's delicious fun either way. The basic method is quite straightforward: you bring yourself or your partner to the "plateau" phase of arousal, where your pleasure is deep and nearing release, and then, just before the genital orgasm sets off its fireworks and explodes everything, you pause, change your method of stimulation. Don't stop entirely, but change pace from fast to slow, or alter the position of your hand. Change, relax, and then carry on pleasing

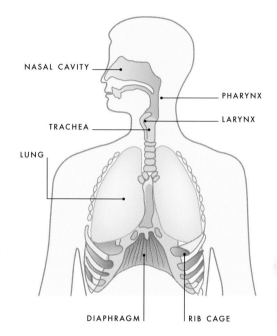

NASAL CAVITY

PHARYNX

LARYNX

TRACHEA

LUNG

DIAPHRAGM

RIB CAGE

Abdominal breathing
Abdominal breathing depends on the diaphragm—the muscle right at the base of the lungs that pulls them up and down. If you're breathing from your diaphragm, you should feel your belly rise and fall.

yourself. It can take a certain amount of experience not to tip over into full-on orgasm—and if you do, remember that you haven't failed, you've just had a delightful experience.

Yogic breathing

A technique that may help you stay
on the edge is yogic breathing. There
are many yogic breathing techniques,
but the abdominal breath is one that's
easy for beginners and goes well with
edging. Try this:

• Place your free hand on your belly,
and try to relax as much of your body
as you can—especially your jaw, face,
and shoulders.

• Exhale, slowly and fully, so your belly
squeezes back toward your spine.

• Take a deep inhalation, feeling your
hand rise as your belly floats upward.

• Repeat this while continuing to pleasure
yourself and hover as close to orgasm as
you possibly can.

This can be a particularly good exercise
for men in heterosexual relationships.
It's not unusual for men to climax sooner
than women, which can leave a female
partner feeling frustrated. The body
learns, though, and the more you practice
delaying an orgasm, the more natural it
will seem—which extends male pleasure
as well as female.

YOGA EXERCISE: CAT-COW
When you want to warm your body up for sex, the cat-cow yoga poses are a great way to release tension and loosen your spine. You can do it as a complete beginner and needn't be especially fit. It's also a sequence that's a lot of fun for a partner to watch!

Cat pose

1 Begin on all fours in a "tabletop" stance, your back straight, your knees placed directly under your hips and your wrists and elbows in a straight line to your shoulders. Keep your head central and not too upright.

2 Exhale, and arch your spine upward like a Halloween cat, making sure your shoulders and knees don't move out of position. Let your head relax down toward the floor.

3 Inhale, returning to your first position. Then move to the Cow pose.

Cow pose

1 Begin in your tabletop position.

2 Inhale. Lift your shoulders and hips toward the ceiling, letting your belly drop down between them. Lift up your head and look forward.

3 Exhale, returning to your tabletop position.

Keep alternating these poses, doing between ten and twenty of each.

TABLETOP POSITION

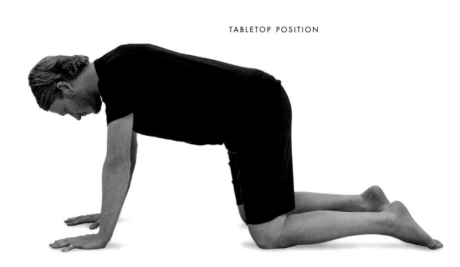

Relax Your Tummy

It's common for many people, especially those of us who feel our stomachs could be more washboard-like than they are, to hold our tummy muscles taut. This is one of those exercises where you should stop worrying about your belly and let it hang loose: cramping it up too much will make it harder for your body to release tension. Let go of your worries and enjoy the stretches.

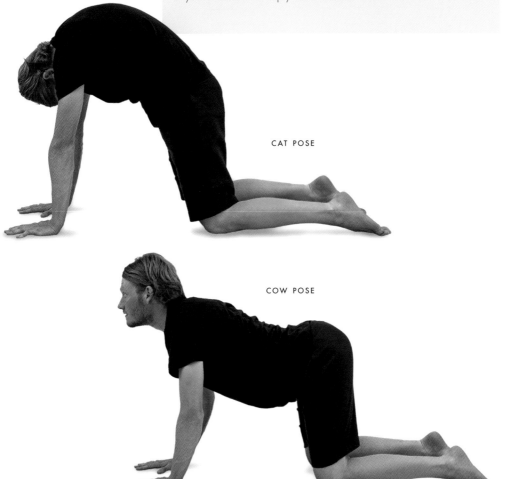

CAT POSE

COW POSE

65

YOGA EXERCISE: DOWNWARD-FACING DOG

The downward-facing dog is a classic yoga pose that strengthens and stretches the limbs. If you work at a desk, it's also a great way to unlock your back and chest, which should help you with deep breathing.

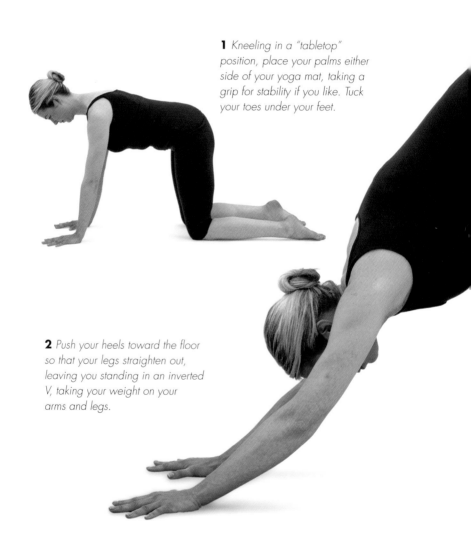

1 *Kneeling in a "tabletop" position, place your palms either side of your yoga mat, taking a grip for stability if you like. Tuck your toes under your feet.*

2 *Push your heels toward the floor so that your legs straighten out, leaving you standing in an inverted V, taking your weight on your arms and legs.*

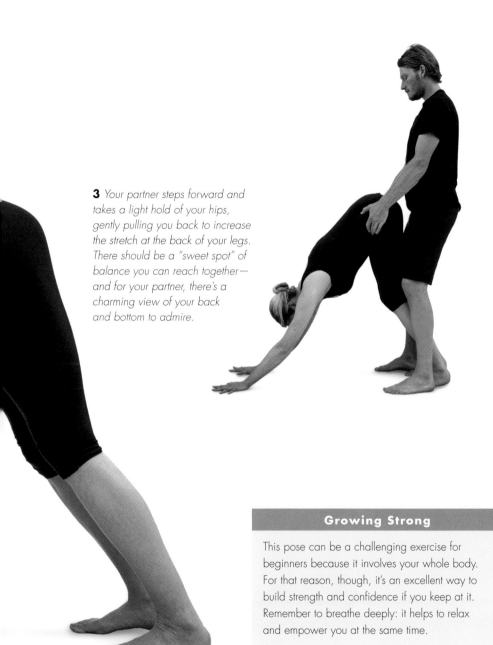

3 *Your partner steps forward and takes a light hold of your hips, gently pulling you back to increase the stretch at the back of your legs. There should be a "sweet spot" of balance you can reach together— and for your partner, there's a charming view of your back and bottom to admire.*

Growing Strong

This pose can be a challenging exercise for beginners because it involves your whole body. For that reason, though, it's an excellent way to build strength and confidence if you keep at it. Remember to breathe deeply: it helps to relax and empower you at the same time.

YOGA EXERCISE: BOUND-ANGLE POSE

The bound-angle pose helps to loosen the hips and strengthen the back—marvelous for anyone planning to wrap themselves around a lover. As a couple, you can also do this exercise facing each other: it's a good position to mix with a gazing meditation (see pages 98–99).

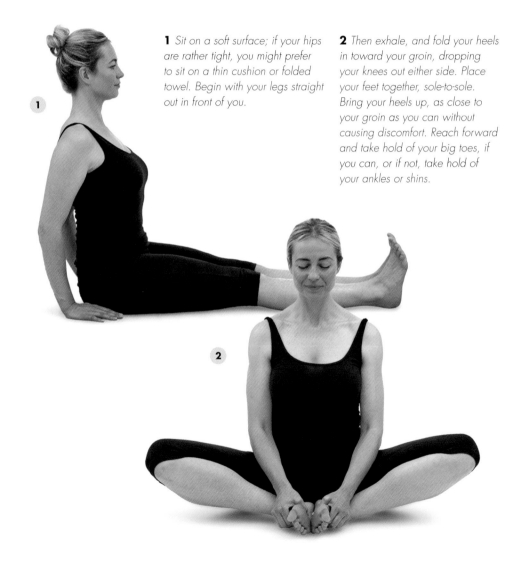

1 *Sit on a soft surface; if your hips are rather tight, you might prefer to sit on a thin cushion or folded towel. Begin with your legs straight out in front of you.*

2 *Then exhale, and fold your heels in toward your groin, dropping your knees out either side. Place your feet together, sole-to-sole. Bring your heels up, as close to your groin as you can without causing discomfort. Reach forward and take hold of your big toes, if you can, or if not, take hold of your ankles or shins.*

Stop When You Are Ready

Don't feel that you and your partner have to stop at the same time: the idea is to love each other's unique selves, not try to become the same. Whichever person wants to stop first can just sit with their legs extended forward until the other is ready to join them.

3 Relax into a balanced position so that your perineum is level with the floor. Don't try to force your legs more "open" than they naturally want to fall: just let gravity do the work.

4 Breathe deeply, letting your chest be open and upright, and rest in this pose for a few minutes.

5 When you've had enough, lift your knees upward, and extend your legs forward again, back into your starting position.

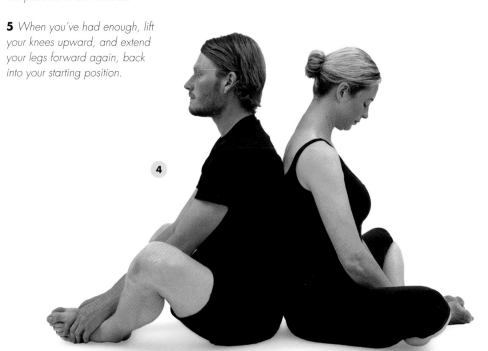

4

YOGA EXERCISE: WIDE-ANGLE SEATED FORWARD BEND

Like the bound-angle pose on the previous page, this is an exercise that can be done facing a lover. You may like to brace your back against a wall to make sure you stay upright—if you both need to brace, you can take turns and the lover away from the wall can do a bound-angle pose instead. This exercise releases the groin and stretches the backs of the legs, making you able to try many sexual positions more easily.

1 *Sitting cross-legged on a mat or blanket, rest your fingertips on the floor next to your hips. From here, place your legs wide apart. Exactly how wide you can comfortably go will be an individual matter: set them far enough apart that you feel a stretch, but not so far that you feel serious pain. Remember, you'll be able to stretch further the more you practice.*

2 *Set the backs of your thighs firmly against the floor, making sure that your knees and toes are facing the ceiling. Stretch from your groin, pushing your heels forward and drawing the balls of your feet upward. Don't let your heels leave the floor, as this will strain your knee joints; just lengthen your legs along the ground.*

3 *Press your fingertips to the floor and take a few deep breaths, lifting your back, ribs, and chest gently upward, which should loosen your back.*

4 *If you already feel fairly stretched, stay in this pose and let your muscles ease into it. There's no need to push yourself: you should feel challenged, but not seriously uncomfortable. If, however, you feel you could stretch more, bend forward by tilting your pelvis and hinging from your hips, keeping your back straight. Walk your hands forward in front of you for support until you are as far forward as you can comfortably go. Breathe, and let your spine extend.*

5 *When you feel ready to finish, inhale, and walk your hands back toward your groin to support yourself as you straighten up. Place them back next to your hips, take another deep breath, and release the pose.*

Be Gentle with Yourself

Some of us have naturally bendy bodies, but for others, these exercises can take some getting used to. Remember, your body is precious no matter what it's like, so if you start off a bit stiff, don't judge yourself harshly. Most importantly, don't push to the point where the stretch is genuinely painful. There's a chance you could injure yourself, and it's hardly good for sexual delight to teach yourself to associate these exercises with feeling sore and uncomfortable. Do what feels right to you: the point is to become better in your body, not worse!

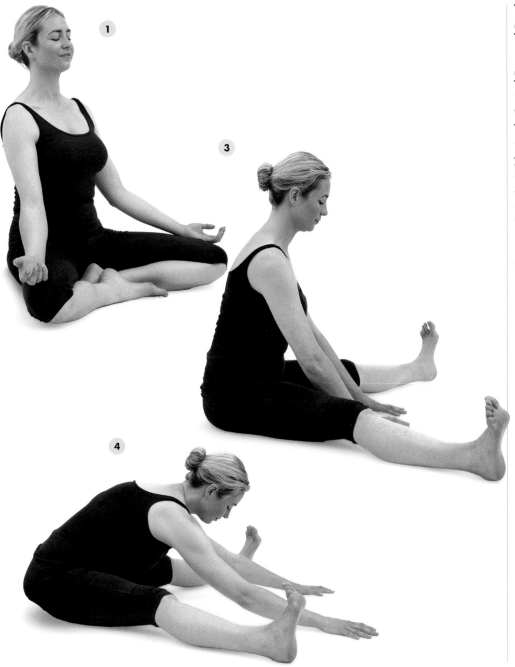

YOGA EXERCISE: WARRIOR POSE

Sex can take stamina, and the Warrior pose is excellent for building up our strength and endurance. This pose is known as Warrior II, and also as Virabhadra, which is a fierce incarnation of Shiva, pictured as having a thousand eyes, hands, feet, and clubs, and wearing a tiger skin. If you want to feel vigorous, this is the position for you.

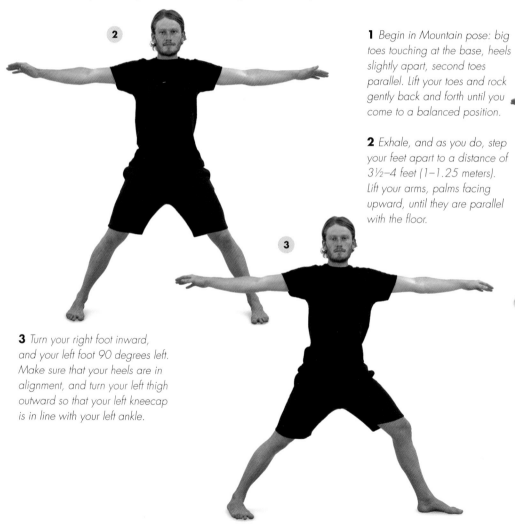

1 *Begin in Mountain pose: big toes touching at the base, heels slightly apart, second toes parallel. Lift your toes and rock gently back and forth until you come to a balanced position.*

2 *Exhale, and as you do, step your feet apart to a distance of 3½–4 feet (1–1.25 meters). Lift your arms, palms facing upward, until they are parallel with the floor.*

3 *Turn your right foot inward, and your left foot 90 degrees left. Make sure that your heels are in alignment, and turn your left thigh outward so that your left kneecap is in line with your left ankle.*

Protect Your Knees

This is a pose that requires both flexibility and strength to hold steady, so make sure you keep your knees in a good position. Knee and foot should be pointed in the same direction with no twisting, the one balanced over the other.

5

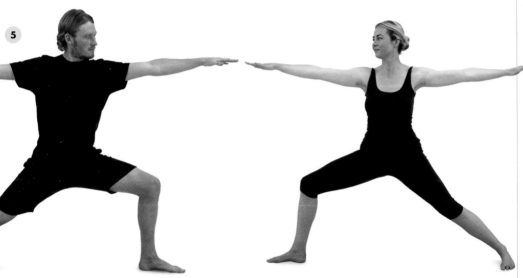

4 *Exhale, and lean to the side, bending your left knee over your left ankle so that your shin is at right angles to the floor. Keep your right leg solid and your outer right heel firmly grounded.*

5 *Stretch your arms outward, still parallel to the floor, opening the space between your shoulder blades. Your torso should be balanced and upright, not leaning to the left, and your shoulders should be in line with your hips. Turn your head to the left and look out past your hand—perhaps into your lover's eyes.*

6 *Stay in this pose for 30 seconds to a minute. When you feel ready, inhale and come gently up. Repeat for the other side of your body.*

YOGA EXERCISE: HAPPY BABY POSE

A good pose to stretch the groin and spine, this is one that can be done as a couple. Having a partner to help you creates face-to-face intimacy, and is also great for beginners who might have trouble keeping a grip on their feet. Best of all, this pose helps you communicate through pressure and counter-pressure, creating the kind of physical conversation that's at the heart of good sex.

1 *Lie on your back and, exhaling, bend your knees up toward your chest. If your stomach is fairly flat, you can do this easily; if you have a pad of flesh there, part your legs so that they rest either side of it.*

2 *Have your partner take hold of your feet and, with an inhalation, open your knees to slightly further apart than the width of your torso. Your partner then leans carefully forward and brings them up toward your armpits. If you're the guiding partner, remember, don't lean too much weight on the legs; just steer them into a comfortable position.*

3 *With your shins perpendicular to the floor and directly above your knees, push your heels gently up against your partner's hands. This is a dance of friendly resistance: there should be enough for you to feel the push, but not enough to make a struggle.*

4 *When you're ready, let your partner know, and drop your legs back to the floor again.*

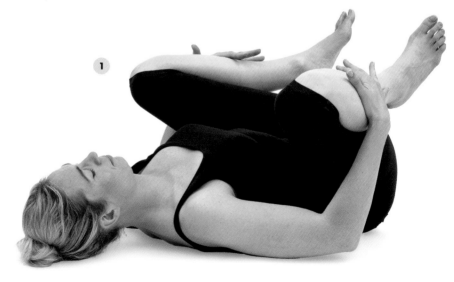

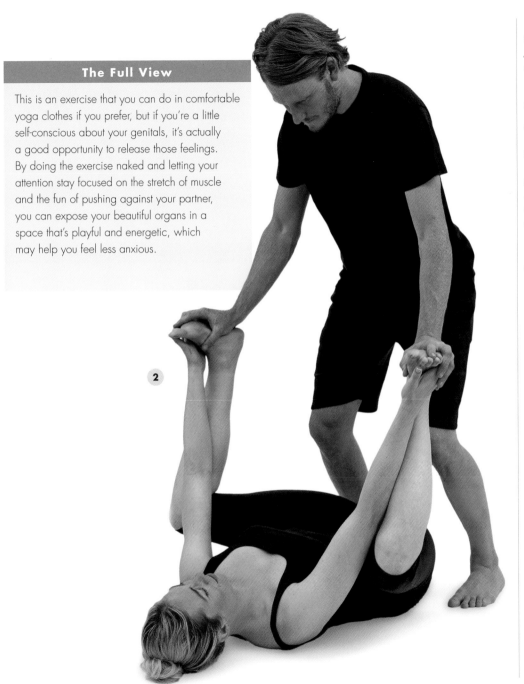

The Full View

This is an exercise that you can do in comfortable yoga clothes if you prefer, but if you're a little self-conscious about your genitals, it's actually a good opportunity to release those feelings. By doing the exercise naked and letting your attention stay focused on the stretch of muscle and the fun of pushing against your partner, you can expose your beautiful organs in a space that's playful and energetic, which may help you feel less anxious.

2

YOGA EXERCISE: BOAT POSE This is a practice that can be done

solo, but it's a lot of fun to do as a couple: your bodies support each other and there's plenty of space for eye-to-eye gazing. You can create a balance between the two of you that's both solid and playful—exactly what you want in a Tantric sexual relationship.

1 *Sit nearly opposite each other on the floor. Begin with your legs straight out in front of you. Then to get the right distance, shift closer to let your legs flow past each other and line your whole bodies at a slight angle to each other rather than twisting your spines.*

2 *Press your hands to the floor a little behind your hips, palms flat and fingers pointing forward. Lean back slightly, lifting from your chest and making sure your back stays flat and straight, creating a three-pointed "tripod" between your tailbone and the tops of your thighbones.*

3 *Exhaling, bend your knees, lift your feet off the floor to an angle of about 45–50 degrees, and rest your feet against your partner's.*

4 *Now straighten your legs if you can, but keep them bent if you can't. The two of you are creating a "W" shape. If you can, stretch your arms along your legs, parallel to the floor, and reach strongly forward through your fingers. This takes some balance and strength, as well as an equally stable partner, so don't do it unless you feel confident. At first, it can help to hold hands with your partner as you practice this, then let go and touch fingertips as you build in confidence.*

5 *At first, don't expect to be able to maintain this pose for more than about ten seconds, but you can build up your times gradually. When you're ready to stop, lower your legs on an exhalation and sit upright on an inhalation, and embrace.*

Soft Landing

Make sure you're somewhere soft, so that it's all right to collapse in a giggling heap if necessary—which, as far as Tantric sex goes, is a perfectly good outcome.

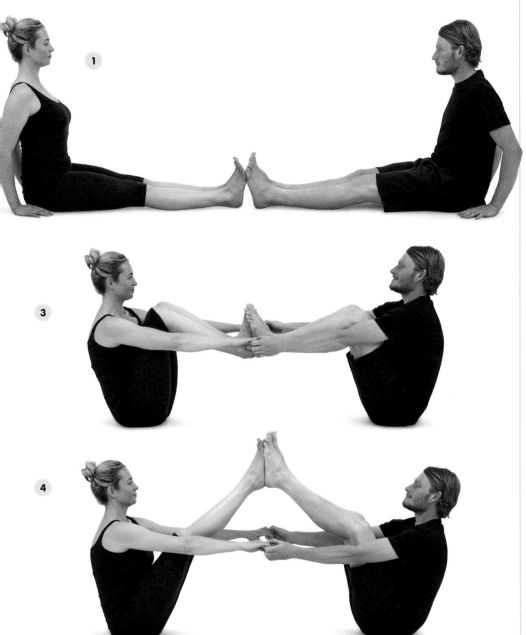

The PC & BC Muscles

A long with spiritual concepts like chakras, good Tantric sex includes an understanding of some anatomy. If you haven't heard of the pubococcygeus muscle, it's time to meet one of the most useful sexual organs you possess.

refer to as your "pelvic floor," and it's through the PC muscle that we're able to open and close the urethra, anus, and vagina. It's the strength of the PC muscle that powers the muscles that contract when we experience orgasm.

The PC muscle

The PC muscle is basically a hammock, one that supports the base of your abdomen and runs from the coccyx, or tailbone, all along the bottom of the pelvic cavity. It's the muscle doctors

The BC muscle

When it comes to the penis, there's another muscle that plays a key role: the bulbocavernosus or BC muscle. Its two main roles are squeezing more blood into the penis, and squeezing semen (or urine)

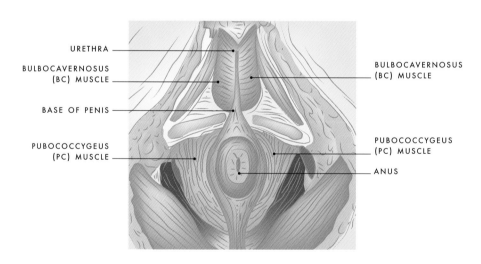

URETHRA

BULBOCAVERNOSUS
(BC) MUSCLE

BASE OF PENIS

PUBOCOCCYGEUS
(PC) MUSCLE

BULBOCAVERNOSUS
(BC) MUSCLE

PUBOCOCCYGEUS
(PC) MUSCLE

ANUS

Male PC and BC muscles

For men, the PC muscle and BC muscle work together to support erections and ejaculations.

out. For this reason, then, a healthy BC muscle is a great asset, as it powers both a firm erection and a strong ejaculation.

In traditional Tantric terminology, these are muscles you'd find around your root chakra (see page 38). The old masters knew whereof they spoke when they associated that chakra with our deepest impulses, because modern anatomists agree that these parts of our body are crucial to our sexual functioning.

How do we know when we have those muscles tensed? The simplest way is to squeeze the part of yourself you'd use to stop yourself urinating. (Don't actually try to stop your urine mid-flow; urologists advise that this can cause health problems.) Tense those muscles up, and you've found your PC and BC.

Exercising the PC and BC muscles is just as helpful for a good sex life as yogic stretches, if not more so. A strong pelvic floor can help support and sustain arousal, allowing us to luxuriate in those delicious sensations for as long as we choose.

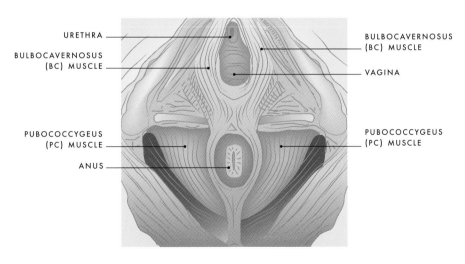

URETHRA

BULBOCAVERNOSUS (BC) MUSCLE

BULBOCAVERNOSUS (BC) MUSCLE

VAGINA

PUBOCOCCYGEUS (PC) MUSCLE

PUBOCOCCYGEUS (PC) MUSCLE

ANUS

Female PC and BC muscles

For women, the PC muscle is the main player in orgasms and pelvic floor control.

Root Exercises for the Vulva

The "pelvic floor"—by which we mostly mean the pubococcygeus (PC) muscle—is central to a healthy sex life. Some twentieth-century exercises known as "Kegels" are your best guide here.

In 1948, an American gynecologist named Dr. Arthur Kegel published an article explaining how women might, without surgical intervention, restore their pelvic floor after childbirth. Whether you've had a baby or not, these are the exact exercises you need to strengthen your root chakra muscles.

Exercise anywhere

You can do Kegel squeezes anywhere—on the bus, in a boring meeting, having coffee with your neighbor. However, to introduce yourself, try it as a meditation.

Sit down somewhere comfortable, breathe mindfully, and send an Inner Smile (see page 30) to your vagina and pelvic floor.

Squeeze your PC muscle. Remember, don't tense any other muscles: if you find yourself rising because your legs are clenching, or your stomach is knotting, relax. Don't hold your breath: breathe calmly. It may feel weak at first, but you

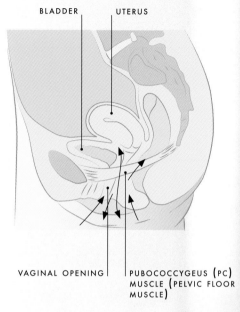

BLADDER   UTERUS

VAGINAL OPENING | PUBOCOCCYGEUS (PC) MUSCLE (PELVIC FLOOR MUSCLE)

Kegel squeeze

The exercise pulls up all the muscles through your vagina, perineum, and anal area. Kegel squeezes are very discreet, so you can practice them wherever you please.

can build it. Squeeze and hold for a count of five seconds, then release. Do this as many times as you can—start with five, perhaps, and then build up from there.

Squeeze rapidly, as many times as you can. Again, you can start with a few and build up. When you're ready, take some deep breaths, smile broadly, relax, and open your eyes.

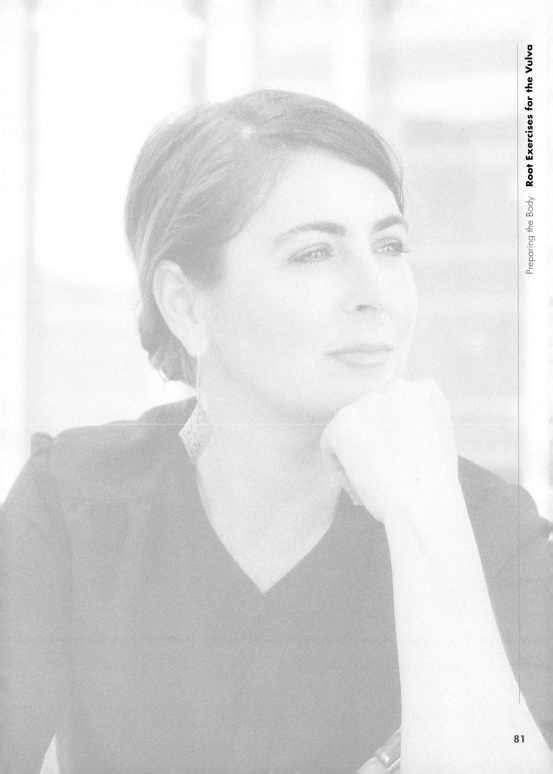

Root Exercises for the Penis

If you have a penis, you'll be working both your pubococcygeus (PC) and bulbocavernosus (BC) muscles here. Don't worry too much about which you're targeting, as they work together and the exercises will strengthen both: just think of it as the broad muscle group that powers your erections and ejaculations.

Core strengthening

While pelvic floor exercises have been recommended for women, especially women post-childbirth, since the mid-twentieth century, more recent research has been encouraging those of us with penises and testicles to enjoy the benefits as well. When your penis is flaccid, use the basic practice on the previous page. The experience is slightly different from those with a vagina, as you'd expect, but the meaning is the same: you are honoring your sexual base, your strong core that underpins your pleasures. They can help you have a stronger sexual center, more control over your erections, and more powerful ejaculations.

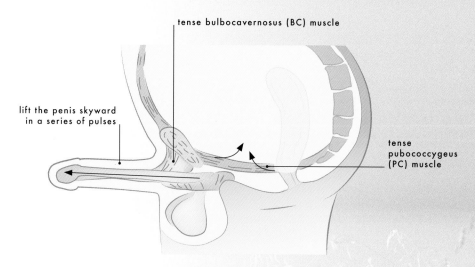

tense bulbocavernosus (BC) muscle

lift the penis skyward in a series of pulses

tense pubococcygeus (PC) muscle

Muscular foundation
A few minutes of exercising every day can give your penis a powerful muscular foundation.

Fun twist

After building yourself up for a few weeks of this, there's a fun twist you can do with your partner:

• Naked and happy, embrace, caress, and play with your partner until you're fully erect.

• Sitting down or standing up—the angle of your erection will be your main guide to which is best for you—ask your partner to extend their hand out, an inch or two above your penis.

• By tensing your PC and BC muscles, flick your penis upward to tap their hand in a merry dance of greeting.

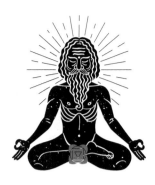

Root chakra

This is an exercise that allows you to enjoy both your own root chakra and your partner's. You are embracing each other on the most primal level.

PC PRACTICE WITH YOUR PARTNER

A good PC and root chakra practice is a fine habit to incorporate into your daily routine, but as with so much about sex, it's delightful to do it with another person. You and your partner can be a warm source of encouragement and pleasure when it comes to keeping your muscles toned. There's nothing that makes an exercise regime more pleasant than mixing in some fondling. As you and your partner work on this technique, you can enjoy being the other's helper and lover at the same time.

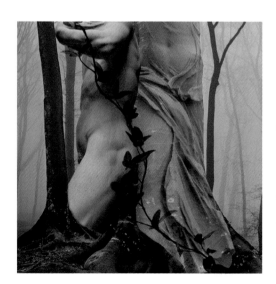

The intimacy of nurture

We all need caring from our partner. The best kind of relationship is where we love our partner's well-being as well as what they can offer us: by helping each other with PC practice, we are giving each other the gift of stronger bodies as well as physical pleasure.

1 *Sit between your lover's legs, and gently place your hand in the place where you'll feel their PC muscles. The perineum—the part that runs between the base of the penis and the anus—is good, or else you can slip two fingers inside your lover's vagina.*

2 *Your lover now begins their clenching exercises. You should be able to feel the muscles tighten and relax against your hand.*

3 *Encourage your partner by giving rewarding little caresses and teases every time they finish a round of repetitions. If this turns into lovemaking, all the better: you can practice the PC clenches one more way—by tightening your vagina around, or flexing your penis inside, your lover.*

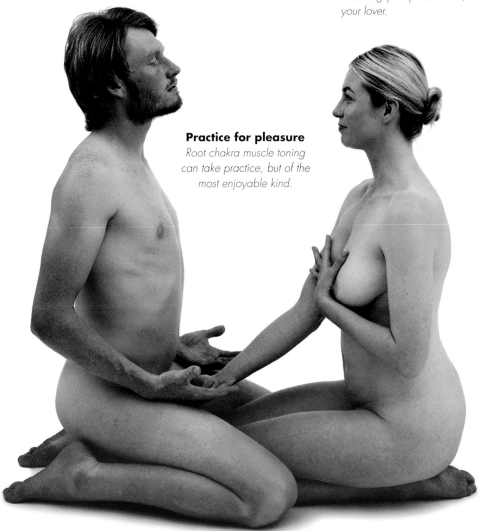

Practice for pleasure
Root chakra muscle toning can take practice, but of the most enjoyable kind.

PREPARING THE PARTNERSHIP

We are all part of the universal bliss. That includes you, and it includes whoever you choose to be your lover. The reason we have sex is to create an intimate physical exchange with another soul, housed in another body. This doesn't mean that you can only have Tantric sex with "the One"; go about it with respect and kindness and you can have Tantric sex with any willing person you like. What it does mean is that, within the sexual space, we have to treat each other as precious—as creatures both utterly unique and entirely part of the vast vibrant universe, entirely ourselves and entirely part of a greater whole. We can do this in a lifelong partnership or a short fling, so long as while we're with someone, we're *with* them: prepared to focus on our mutual delight in each other and give the experience our full attention.

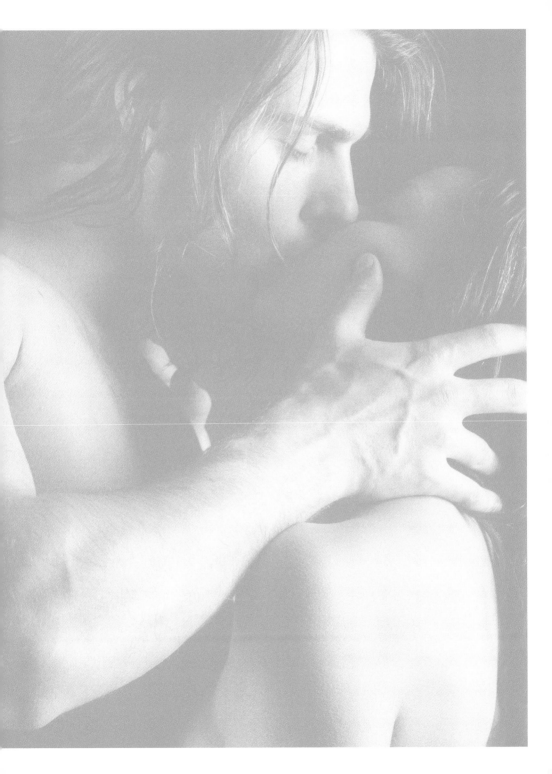

The Harmonious Couple

Connecting with a lover is one of the most blissful and most vulnerable things in the world. We yearn for it—and yet, it can seem complicated. Tantric sex can be a simple, yet subtle, resolution of the paradox.

In the glow of a new relationship, everything seems possible, but we fear failure: will our beloved still want us when they discover our imperfections? In a long-established relationship, we feel as if we know each other well, but we fear disenchantment: when we share the mundane work of everyday life, can we still be thrilling and mysterious to each other?

Body and soul

Tantric sex says yes. What we need in a relationship with a lover is the same thing we need in a relationship with ourselves: acceptance, faith, and compassion.

The human psyche is a fluid thing. Buddhists might say we have no real "self"—or at least, no set-in-stone, unchanging identity. Our feelings change moment to moment, and our character adapts as we learn and develop. When we love another person, we aren't loving a single set of traits: we're loving a process, as constant, and yet as capable of surprise, as we ourselves.

When we undertake a Tantric relationship, we may feel that we're going to transform ourselves. This is true in a way, but the way we do this is by *not trying to change each other*. Just as suffering comes from refusing to accept that the world changes and is never quite within our control, the same can be said of relationships.

Communication

Of course, this doesn't mean you can never ask for more help with the dishes or point out that a careless remark hurt your feelings. Communicating our needs is fundamental to a healthy relationship. What it means is that to come together in harmony, we need to approach each other with a fundamental acceptance. Joy in our partner isn't something we create, it's something we notice has always been there—or at least, was always ready for us to feel the moment we accepted it.

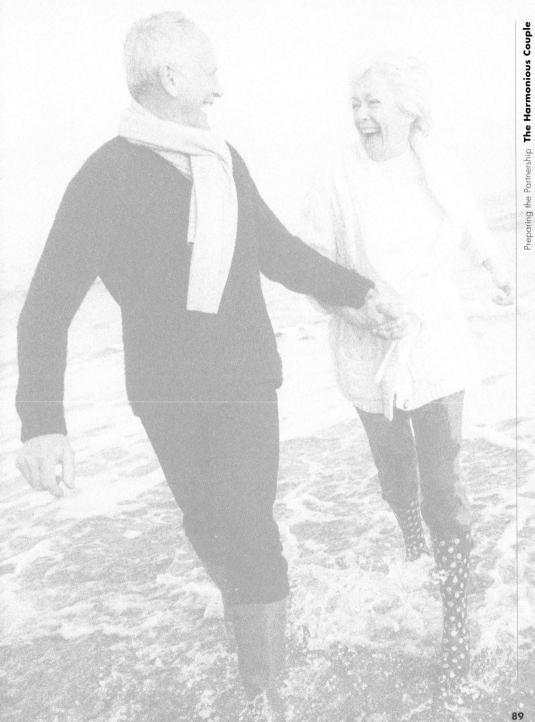

The Qualities of a Good Partner

We all dream of Mr. or Ms. Right. In Tantra, there's really no such thing as "right" or "wrong"—everything that is, is—but there are certainly ways of being that can make your relationship flow better.

In opening yourself to Tantric sex, you are lowering your guard. The experiences can throw up deep emotions, strong sensations, memories and hopes, and confusions and fears that you might not have expected. If you and your lover are setting out on this voyage, you need to be able to trust each other. Cultivate the following qualities in yourself, and hold out for a partner who's prepared to give them to you.

Respect

Sacred sex is done by sacred bodies and spirits, and for that to work, you need to appreciate each other's needs and rights. You don't have to agree on everything—for some couples, a little difference is the spice of life—but you must feel that your lover sees you as a good, reasonable, and interesting human being who deserves to be heard. You will be learning from each other, so respect each other as both student and teacher.

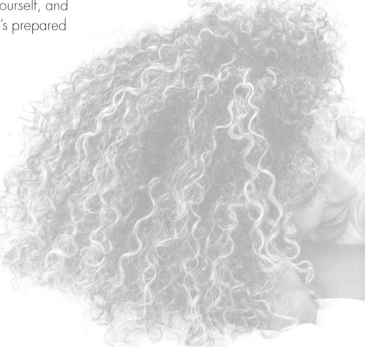

Trust

Nothing distracts from ecstasy like feeling that our partner won't catch us if we fall. Everyone makes mistakes, so a lover doesn't have to be infallible, but make sure you each know that you sincerely intend to stand by each other and treat vulnerabilities with kindness.

Openness

To please a partner, we have to know what pleases them. Tantric sex involves exploring different ways of being, as well as revealing very private truths: partners need to be open to new experiences, and comfortable with the intimacy that goes with telling each other what they're really thinking and feeling.

A partner who's truly unwilling to try these things is shutting themselves off from the bliss that Tantric sex can offer—but Tantric sex can also help to build them. Give yourselves to the experience, and let it connect you.

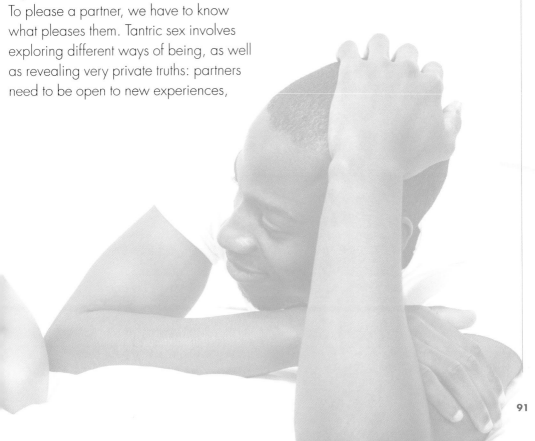

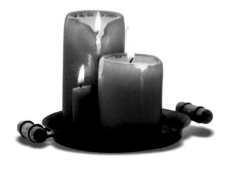

Scent the air

Traditionally, rituals involve incense and lighting candles. A scented candle can be an excellent combination for the space-conscious.

THE SACRED SEXUAL SPACE

Ideally, we should set aside a place in our home purely for sexual spirituality, but it needn't be a dedicated room. Few of us live in houses big enough for that. We just need to be resourceful, and flexible in our thinking: even a spruced-up bedroom can be made sacred.

The sacred space is at once physical and psychological—you create a place to be so you can enter a mental state—so tailor your space to your own psyche and fill it with things that carry meaning to you.

Comfortable
Make it clean and tidy. You'll be rolling and dancing around here, so make every surface touch-friendly.

Focused
Remove any clutter that might distract you, or impede you if you want to dance or try a new sexual position.

Glowing
The light should be soft and welcoming. Candlelight is a favorite. A tip here:

we can become careless in ecstasy, so place them safely out of reach, and favor candles with wide bases or in jars, which are harder to knock over.

Empowering
Traditional sexual spaces can include icons, but you may prefer to choose objects that are iconic to you. If you want to feel grounded, include a sculpture made of solid rock, for instance, or if you want to feel beautiful, add a vase of your favorite flowers. Let your imagination be the guide here.

Sensual
Scent the air; choose a good mattress; have the temperature right. Make it a place where your body feels good.

Quality sheets

Your bed will be the center of your space, so treat yourself to good-quality sheets that feel and look enticing.

Sensual imagery

If your sacred space has to double as a regular bedroom, choose pictures that evoke aspects of your sexuality. If you want to feel part of nature, for instance, choose a natural image: it won't suggest anything to visitors, but you'll know what it means.

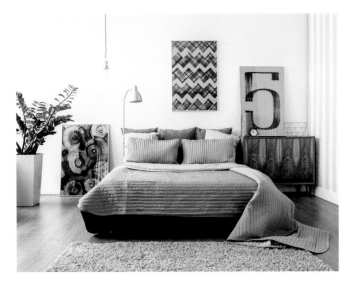

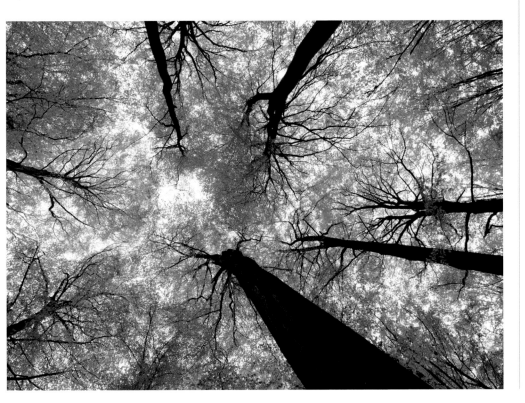

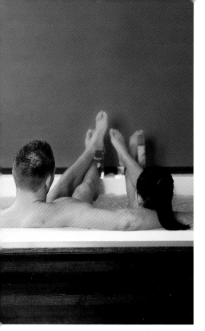

Clean loving

Enter your sacred space clean and scented—you may even like to bathe together.

ENTERING THE SACRED SPACE

Now you have your bedroom or other space set up, how do you approach it? First, let's shed an illusion: your sacred space doesn't need to be "perfect," any more than you do. The only rules are to be open to love and pleasure.

So, how do we enter our space? To begin, it's nice to prepare for the moment. A clean lover is a delicious lover, so bathe first, and enjoy it. Use fine-smelling soap, have a relaxing bath or an invigorating shower, and prepare your body as you'd tune up a fine instrument before playing a duet.

Next, consider dressing the part. You can have ecstatic sex wearing any old rags, or indeed nothing at all, but it's a delightful ritual to prepare. Sleek and loose garments such as an easily-shed robe are excellent. Alternatively, you can tease your imagination and dress as some sexy figure you've always longed to be, whether it's a divine goddess or a naughty nurse—play and fun are good things. Don't limit yourself to one style; you are an endlessly changing and flexible spirit, after all. The only consistent rule should be that whatever you wear is comfortable and can, when the moment is right, be removed easily.

Once you enter, relax and breathe deeply. You are leaving the rest of the world behind: here, you are with yourself and with your lover, and you don't have to worry about anything else.

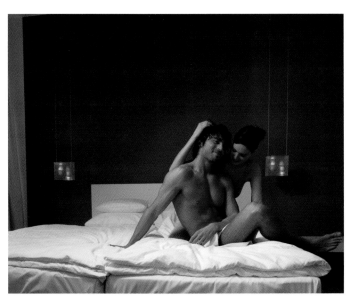

Safe space

The sacred space is private and safe. Leave your worries outside: when you're here, you're here.

Dress the part

Choose garments that feel good to wear and that can be shed without difficulty.

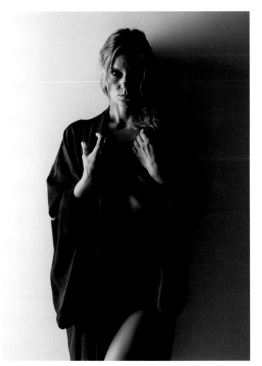

The Sacredness of Joy

The words "sacred space" may sometimes sound a little daunting, especially if you've grown up in a religious tradition that conflates "sacred" with "serious." In a way, what you are doing is serious—but that doesn't mean it has to be a solemn space. Tantra is about transcendence and delight, so don't let the idea of a sacred space alarm you. You go in there to enjoy yourself.

Honoring the Partner

Sacred sex means a sacred partner. That sacredness doesn't come from their being "better" than anyone else, but from their inherent humanity—and from how we choose to treat them.

There are some basic sexual ethics that every reasonable belief system includes, and now, as we begin exploring intimacy, is a good time to examine them and put them in a Tantric context.

Consent

First: a partner's consent must be inviolate. You are creating sexual magic together: do not introduce an impure alloy into that alchemy. Consent obviously means that you mustn't physically force anyone, but it can also be subtler than that. Pestering, pressuring, and manipulating also disregard your partner's consent; so does sulking or complaining if they give you an unwanted "no." By all means seduce and entice, but in the understanding that you must both feel joyful about your experience. If your partner seems not to be feeling that joy, stop at once and create an emotional sacred space where they can say what they're honestly feeling.

Honor your lover's body

Second: a partner's physical health is your sacred duty. For your own sake it's always sensible to take safe sex precautions, but you can also see it as honoring your partner's body. There's nothing unromantic or unspiritual about having the all-important discussion about precautions. On the contrary, you are embracing sex in all its reality—and the reality is that it can, as well as creating ecstasy, create pregnancies and disease transmission. We live in a yin-and-yang world, remember (see pages 44–45), and these things are part of a whole. In Tantric sex, we accept what is, so accept that sex can have unwanted consequences and mindfully prepare to protect yourself and your lover.

These may seem like strictures, but actually it's better to think of them like the framework of a trampoline. If they're solid, we can leap to dizzying heights because we know they're there underneath us, steady and safe. Know your partner's boundaries and needs, and consult a doctor when necessary. You aren't straying outside the sacred space: you're making it possible.

GAZING MEDITATION

Nothing is more intimate than eye contact. When we look at the world around us, only two groups regularly stare right into each others eyes: mothers and babies—and lovers. To gaze at and with your partner is to enter a deep and powerful space.

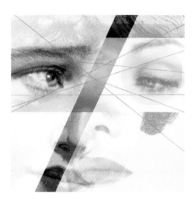

Eye to eye
Look into your lover's eyes, and see deep into possibility.

1 *Sit opposite your partner in a comfortable place, and set a timer for five minutes—preferably one that will sound an alarm that's pleasant rather than startling. Facing each other, set the timer running, close your eyes, and breathe mindfully. Be aware of your own body, and also the sound of breath going in and out of your partner.*

2 *Open your eyes and gaze into your lover's eyes. Just sit and look at each other: you don't have to smile, speak, or do anything except look, and let whatever feelings come up pass through you.*

3 *After five minutes, reach out. Take your partner's hand, then both of you close your eyes and breathe mindfully again for five minutes. This grounds you in a peaceful mental state without breaking the connection.*

Eye Contact

Eye contact can throw up some difficult emotions—because, unaccompanied by complete trust, a stare is usually associated with a challenge or a threat. "Who do you think you're looking at?" people demand as they pick a fight; "Don't you eyeball me!" a superior shouts at an underling—and to avoid trouble, the victim drops their eyes. Prolonged gazing is an experience that can, at first, feel uncomfortable. Which is, of course, one of the main reasons that it's such a thrilling experience—and why, in Tantric sex, we practice it. Being present with each other means removing barriers: to meet each other eye to eye is to create a sexual space in which there is nowhere we can't look.

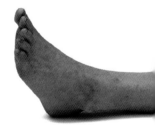

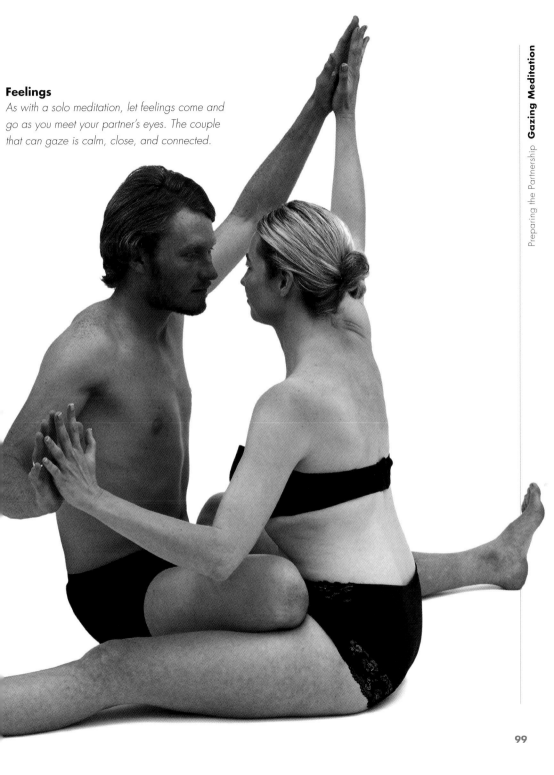

Feelings

As with a solo meditation, let feelings come and go as you meet your partner's eyes. The couple that can gaze is calm, close, and connected.

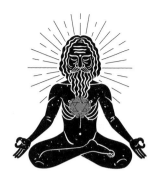

Heart chakra
This is the chakra of balance; by creating a flow between your heart chakra and your partner's, you are extending the balance between you.

LOVERS' GREETING RITUAL
Tantric sex is both calm and exciting. When you're preparing for lovemaking with your partner, let your energy greet theirs: in this way, you start to form the connection that will build to ecstasy.

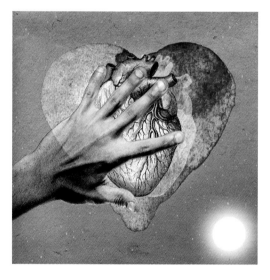

1 *Sit opposite each other in a comfortable position. Look into each other's eyes.*

2 *Begin to work up some Inner Smile energy (see pages 30–31). With a gentle smile, keep gazing at your partner's face and send them your positive will.*

3 *Place your right hand over your head, while your partner does the same. With your left hands, reach out and gently lay them on top of your partner's right hand.*

4 *Begin to feel a flow of energy: a glow is rising through each of your heart chakras (see page 38) and creating a warm circuit between the two of you. Sit like this for a few minutes, creating a flow of energy and positivity.*

Connection
The hands, arms, and lungs are as much a part of the heart chakra as the heart itself: they embody our deepest ability to "reach out" to others.

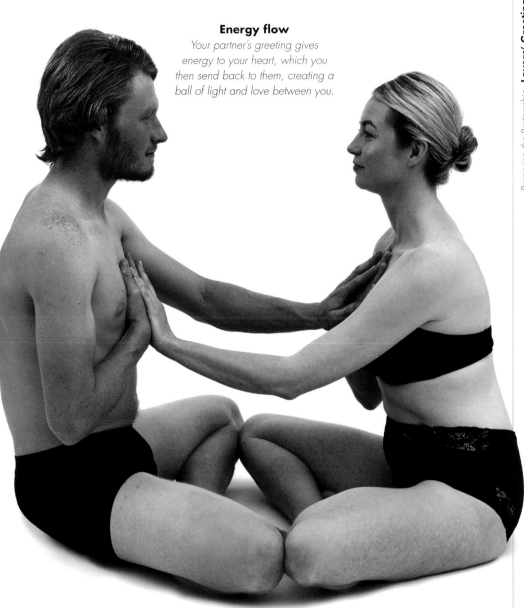

Energy flow
Your partner's greeting gives energy to your heart, which you then send back to them, creating a ball of light and love between you.

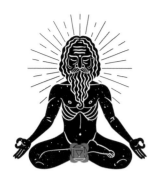

Root chakra
In this chakra rests our ability to feel grounded and part of a community. Be aware of it in this meditation, which helps us feel part of a couple.

HUGGING MEDITATION
The embrace is the foundation of the relationship, both sexual and emotional. Indeed, you and your lover should, on some level, find an embrace in every interaction, be it wrapping your bodies around each other or surrounding each other with a warm glow of acceptance. Any hug is a good hug, but this is a particularly good exercise to repeat before and after lovemaking, deep conversations, meditations, and whenever else you could do with some grounding.

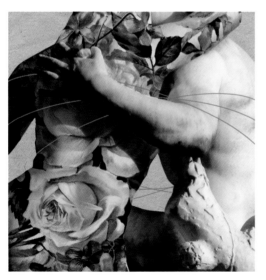

1 *Stand opposite each other. Don't rush together: look into each other's eyes, and then, slowly and tenderly, gaze down the length of your partner's body, right down to the toes, then all the way back up to their face. You are "embracing" their body with your sight.*

2 *Take a deep breath and feel the energy in your root chakra (see page 38). A hug is very primal, so be aware of your primal chakra.*

Intimate embrace
Sex, fundamentally, involves embracing another person's physical self. No sexual relationship can be fully joyful unless good hugs are built in.

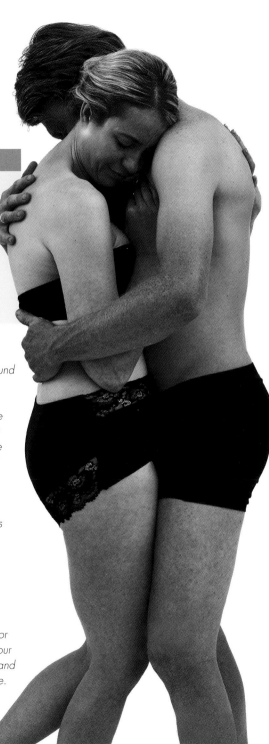

Hugging for Health

Hugs are wonderful. On a physical level, they're actually good for our health, releasing "feel good" hormones such as dopamine and "cuddle" hormones such as oxytocin, making us feel more blissful and bonded to our partners. They're also the perfect way to feel out your intimacy and settle yourselves.

3 *Slowly come together and wrap your arms around each other. Don't squeeze too hard: instead, rest together. Feel every part of your lover's body: the warmth of their skin, the shift of their limbs, the rise and fall of their chest. Open yourself to what their body may be telling you about their emotions: are they leaning in to relax, or carrying any tensions? Flinching any part of themselves away from you? Tentative about touching any part of you? When the hug is finished, you can talk this through, as it can be a way to "feel out" needs that your bodies may be trying to communicate.*

4 *When you're ready, draw a deep breath, step apart, and smile at each other.*

Perfectly imperfect

Worried that your breasts are too small or your tummy is too big? You can't hide your shape in a hug, so take a deep breath and let yourself be welcomed, just as you are.

103

SHARED BREATHING MEDITATION

Breath is life, and as it flows, so flows our energy. What better way to be intimate than to mingle our energy together as one? This is a meditation that's very physically close, so before you begin, make sure you're clean and pleasant to be near. Floss and brush your teeth so you smell good; wash your face; shave off any abrasive stubble or, if you have a beard, condition it a bit so it'll be nice and soft.

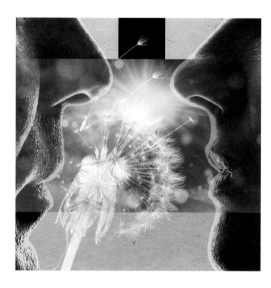

Gentle breath

Let the air caress you in a gentle and stimulating rhythm.

1 *Sit together, one on the other's lap. You might like to sit in the Yab-Yum position (see pages 152–153), but if that's too hard on your legs, one partner sitting on the couch and the other sitting astride is equally good. Settle comfortably together.*

2 *Bring your faces close. Close your eyes and, letting your lips just brush each other, start to breathe together. As one partner inhales, the other exhales. Feel the brush of air over your face, your energy starting to mingle.*

3 *Close your lips together in a sealed kiss, and breathe together more deeply. Inhale the air from your partner's lungs, taking in their energy, then release your breath and energy into them. It's a dance of penetration and receptivity in which you both play each part.*

Don't do step 3 for more than a few minutes, as your oxygen levels will start to drop, and certainly don't push yourself if you start to feel dizzy. Lightly tap your partner on the shoulder, and you can draw apart and either start with a new breath or go back to step 2.

4 *Draw gently apart when you feel ready. Embrace for a few minutes and savor the energy glow you've created between each other.*

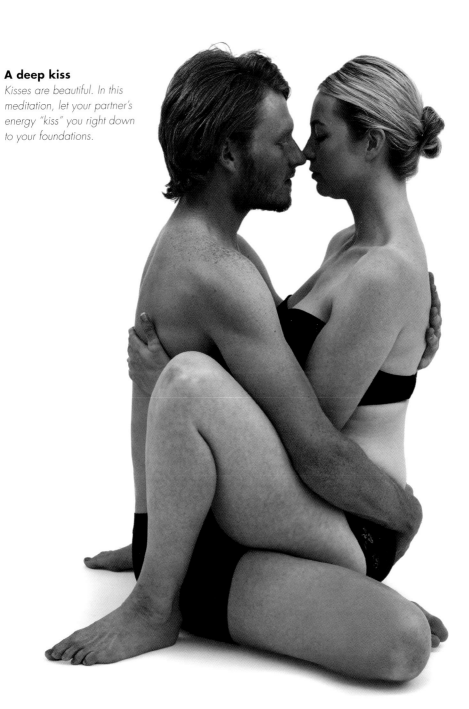

A deep kiss

Kisses are beautiful. In this meditation, let your partner's energy "kiss" you right down to your foundations.

UNDRESSING MEDITATION

Sometimes we have plenty of time to enter the sacred space in the perfect, easy-to-slip-out-of costume—but sometimes we just have to start from where we are. This doesn't mean we can't approach it with Tantric deliciousness, though: it's all in the approach. If you don't have time to change, or else your lover looks so tempting that you just have to get their clothes off now, you can use the Undressing Meditation as a way to settle yourselves into the moment quickly.

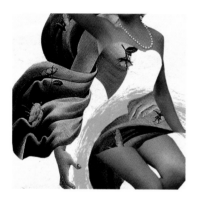

Elegant reality

Are your partner's clothes easy to slip off, or do you have to tug and struggle a bit? It doesn't matter: feel yourself graceful and confident in your every move.

1 *For two minutes, tantalize yourselves. Rest your hands on whatever part of your lover's body you most love to grab—and which is currently being kept from you by a layer or two of fabric. Really focus on the sensation in your hands: the heat of your lover's body seeping through the clothes, the textures of denim or wool that separate you, the folds, pockets, or zippers that baffle your touch, and the gorgeous shape underneath. Gaze into each other's eyes and let your hands yearn in stillness.*

2 *Remove one of your hands and start unzipping or unbuttoning whatever garment is keeping you from that lovely body part. Keep your other hand resting on it. If this feels a little awkward, laugh about it— the challenge and frustration is part of the fun.*

3 *Finally, unpeel the clothing, letting your hand experience the shock of transition from fabric to flesh as you finally come into contact with the desired body part. By now, you've worked up a lot of energy, and you can either repeat the tease with another body part and garment or just tear each other's clothes off and start enjoying each other's naked skin with newly awakened appreciation.*

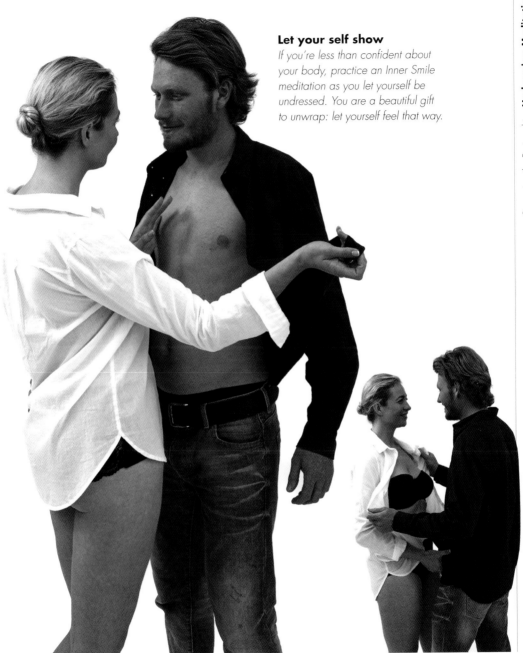

Let your self show

If you're less than confident about your body, practice an Inner Smile meditation as you let yourself be undressed. You are a beautiful gift to unwrap: let yourself feel that way.

CARESSING MEDITATION

We can learn a world of sensations simply by touching our lover and watching, with full and meditative attention, how they respond. This is a thoroughly pleasurable meditation that should be done at the beginning of any new relationship—and, since we change over time, regularly throughout an established one to keep us "in touch" with our partner's feelings and sensations.

1 *In a Caressing Meditation, your partner lies on their front and you stroke them from nape to feet, then back up again.*

2 *Repeat your caress several times. Try varying the pressure you use and the speed at which you move: pay intimate attention to what your partner responds to the most.*

3 *Next they turn over, and you repeat the process on the other side. Be alert and responsive as you feel for the exact balance of touch: you are reading them with your hands.*

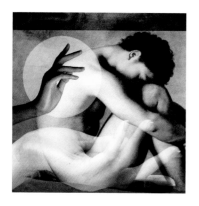

Stroking

Stroke every part of your partner's skin, and do it more than once: the perfect level of pressure will be different depending on whether the touch is new or not.

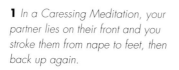

Right or Wrong Touch?

What is the "right" way to touch a partner? The answer is going to vary from individual to individual, and on that individual, from place to place on their body—and even then, it can vary from moment to moment, as our skin grows used to one level of contact and craves something firmer. What we can all agree is that being touched "wrong" isn't sexy. Overly rough contact feels insensitive, and possibly even threatening; overly light touch feels irritating, ticklish, and itchy. The touch we adore occupies the finely balanced point between these extremes—light enough to tantalize us, firm enough to melt us, a touch that's confident and sweet and delectable. How do we find that touch? We practice, and we watch. This is the essence of becoming a fine lover: we learn to read the body of our partner.

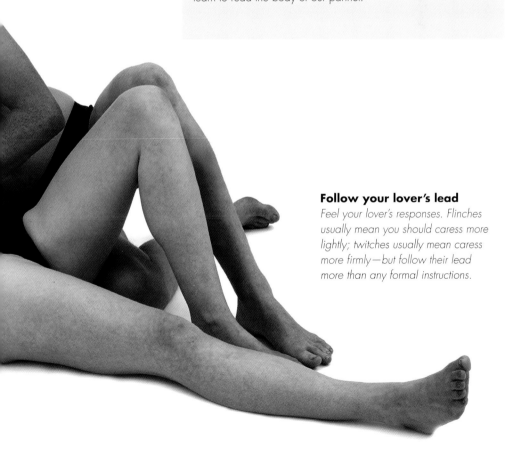

Follow your lover's lead

Feel your lover's responses. Flinches usually mean you should caress more lightly; twitches usually mean caress more firmly—but follow their lead more than any formal instructions.

Playfulness, Silliness & Joy

Because we associate Tantra with ancient wisdom, it's easy to assume that it has to be deadly earnest and serious. The truth is quite different.

One of the great stumbling blocks of the human mind, spiritually speaking, is its tendency to dualistic thinking—something is *either* this *or* it's that. We are either individuals or we're part of a greater whole; we're either physical or spiritual—we're either wise or frivolous. Tantra came along to sweep away such distinctions; dualistic thinking is, in fact, something many religions, including many that have incorporated Tantra, identify as one of the biggest causes of suffering. Consider, for instance, Zen Buddhism's heavy reliance on paradox: apparently silly things can be the path to enlightenment.

Be a wise fool

Think of it this way: of the people you know, are the ones who take themselves very, very seriously and never find a funny side to anything the wisest or most perceptive? Probably not: we should feel compassion for them, as they're likely afraid, but we shouldn't follow their example in the bedroom.

Do you feel silly trying any Tantric exercise? Fine: laugh at yourself. Are you worried you'll look foolish to your partner? Be a wise fool and don't worry about it.

Playful learning

How did you learn when you were a child? You played. You imitated, pretended, spun flights of fancy—and in so doing, connected with other people, discovered your own capacities, acquired skills. The thing about play is that it makes something *safe*: you can afford mistakes, because all that means is that you tumble down, giggle, and get back up. When we feel there's something terribly important at stake, we tend to clam up: it's very hard to take a risk if you aren't relaxed, because the natural response to a threat is to hunker down and stick to what's safe. And what's safe is what we know already.

When we're trying a new world of sensation and exploration, that won't carry us very far. What we're looking for here is joy, and joy doesn't come from perfectionism. Sex isn't supposed to be dignified, and play certainly isn't.

Feel free to be joyfully silly—because then you're free.

The Purity of Dirty Jokes

Should sacred sex be joked about? By all means—as long as you and your partner are comfortable with it. The most important thing is to be sensitive to where your partner's limits are: if you find dirty jokes funny but your partner would rather keep some things joke-free, give them the gift of your respect on that point. The best kind of laughter is where we're free to laugh at ourselves, and we feel most able to do that with partners we know we can trust to stop laughing when we need them to.

LAUGHING MEDITATION

If you can learn to laugh, you're well on your way to bliss: laughter frees the spirit from self-consciousness, not to mention exercising the body and making it stronger and sexier. A good laugh really can be some of the best medicine you can give yourself. You and your partner can try a lovely variation of this. Did you ever play "staring match" as a child, where you and a friend locked eyes and waited to see who would laugh first? A good gazing practice between you and your partner (see Gazing Meditation on pages 98–99) might free you of the self-consciousness that makes laughter near impossible in "staring match," but that doesn't mean you can't also enjoy setting each other off.

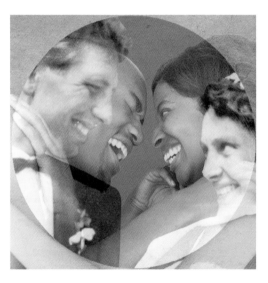

1 *Sit down opposite each other and meet each other's gaze.*

2 *Begin laughing. Now, this may feel artificial at first, but that's all right: just start walking your body through the process.*

3 *Keep looking at each other. Watching another person laugh lifts the spirits, and you can catch a laughing mood off each other—either by sparking off your lover's genuine laughter or, after a while, from the sheer silliness of what you're doing. Laugh together for at least three minutes.*

Playful wisdom
Laughter and wisdom are not opposites: enlightenment knows how to see the funny side.

Monk Meditation

Some Tibetan monks begin every day with a laughing meditation: they wake, and before they open their eyes, they spend a minute stretching and letting every muscle "yawn," then for three solid minutes, give a great big belly laugh.

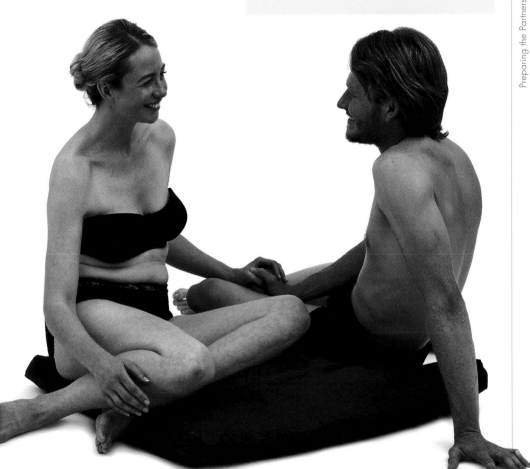

Catch the joy

Catch each other's joyful energy, and you'll be firing each other up, maybe even to the point of a "laughtergasm" (see page 54).

The Spiritual Importance of Equality

Of all the dualities that cloud our minds, one of history's most damaging is the duality between those with power and those without. Tantric practitioners may seek out teachers, but between you and your lover there must always be an acceptance that neither of you is the "superior." Anything else violates the trust between you and your partner, and the honesty of your place within the cosmos.

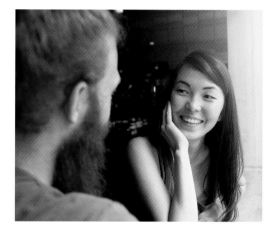

Love without prejudice
The gift you owe your partner is to see them clearly, not through the eyes of a prejudiced world.

Feminine and masculine

Power imbalances can come in many forms. The commonest, in a sexual relationship, is the power imbalance between men and women. While Tantra does usually consider feminine yin and masculine yang as complementary powers (see pages 44–45), it's important to understand that neither dominates the other: each exists as the other's reflection—and in contemporary Tantra, there's no reason to assume that a woman is all yin or a man all yang either (see Gender & Love, pages 116–117). To assume that one partner is the superior simply on the grounds of gender is to be blind to what these symbols really mean.

There are other ways in which you can be imbalanced; after all, we live in an imperfect world. An older partner may have more worldly status and experience than a younger, while the younger may be considered more conventionally attractive by many people, giving potential imbalances on both sides. An inter-racial couple may find that society accords more respect to one of them than the other, calling upon the more advantaged partner to show solidarity and the less advantaged to exercise trust and forgiveness. And some couples simply contain one personality that's more forceful than the other.

Let's be clear: difference can be beautiful, and there is no need to be less than you are, or other than you are, to be part of a relationship. But a superior or domineering partner is not practicing Tantric sex. If there are power differences between you, take the opportunity to see beyond them and recognize them for what they are: the side effects of human mistakes. In Tantric sex, we rise to bliss *together*; we create insight by accepting ourselves and our partners as equals, two parts of the great universe both tiny and infinite.

Gender & Love

Does Tantric sex need a "masculine" man and a "feminine woman"? Not at all. Tantra is about the embrace of opposites—but we all contain enough opposites in ourselves, never mind in a partner, for a lifetime's embrace. Gender is a lot more fluid and slippery than we think, and need be no barrier to Tantric sex.

There's no doubt that in traditional Tantra, male and female archetypes are important. The divine Shiva and his consort Shakti, for instance, are central to Hindu Tantra, while the "feminine" yin and "masculine" yang are important in Taoism.

What's important to understand, though, is that we all contain "masculine" and "feminine" elements.

Focus on qualities not gender

Think of what's traditionally considered "masculine": upright, bold, outgoing, dynamic. Are those admirable traits really qualities that a woman can't have? Will a man somehow magically lose those virtues if he falls in love with another man, or if he happens to be a transsexual man? The idea is ridiculous: look at real people, and they'll disprove it in ten minutes flat. Likewise, what's traditionally "feminine"?

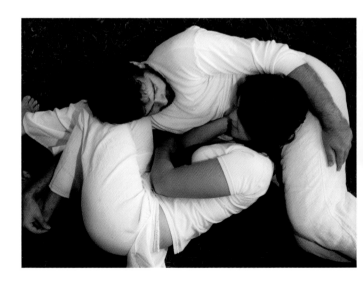

Be open
We all embody both yin and yang. Don't let rigid ideas of gender confuse you: Tantric sex is open to all of us.

Perceptiveness, sensitivity, generosity, warmth—these are qualities that the toughest of manly-men can have in abundance, and are all the better for embracing. "Masculine" and "feminine" are within us all.

Whatever your genders, you contain both yin and yang, and so does your lover. There may be times when you want to express your "yin" side, your receptive or submissive self, and other times when you want to make love in a "yang" state of dominance and action. These are pleasures to be savored: they won't make you less of a man or woman, because being a man or woman isn't about what you do in the bedroom.

Explore

If you find traditional gender roles exciting, then that's just fine: embrace what thrills you. But if you and your lover don't quite fit into the traditional boxes— or if you do, and you'd like to have a peep outside them and see what else you could try—then that's equally valid. Yin and yang are states of mind, not iron-clad gender roles: be open to whatever part of them speaks to and through you.

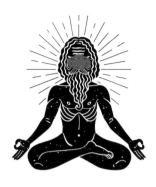

Third-eye chakra
The third-eye chakra is the chakra of intuition and perception, it is the part of our spirit that "sees" the truth.

THIRD-EYE ATTUNEMENT Can we ever see precisely "eye to eye" with our partners? Probably not—accepting our differences is part of Tantric sex—but we can encourage our inner vision to draw closer together. The Third-Eye Attunement meditation is an exercise that symbolizes our commitment to embracing our lover's intuition and understanding.

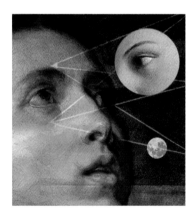

Seeing beyond the surface
There's an old saying that the eyes are the windows of the soul. In this meditation, try experiencing your partner's soul through your energy rather than your sight.

1 *Sit facing opposite each other, as close as you can manage comfortably. If one of you is much taller than the other, the smaller may want to sit on a cushion: you need to be more or less on a level. For a few minutes, close your eyes and relax, sending Inner Smile energy (see pages 30–31) to your third-eye chakra (see page 38).*

2 *When you are ready, open your eyes. Then, lean forward, and gently embrace your partner, bringing your foreheads to rest together. Don't press uncomfortably hard; just come into a position where your third-eye chakras are aligned. Close your eyes again.*

3 *Continue to send Inner Smile energy to this chakra, and as you do, become aware of the heat of your partner's face and the energy at the place where your foreheads are touching. Focus on that place: you are sending energy to the site where your chakras are joined, creating a magic space which isn't quite you or your partner, but a combination of the two.*

4 *After a few minutes, lean forward further, rest your heads on each other's shoulders, and hug for a few minutes to settle your energy. Hug with open awareness of how both your body and your partner's have responded to the experience.*

New insights

In Tantric sex, we are making love to our partner's spirit and mind as well as their body, and in honoring those things, we open ourselves up to new insights of our own.

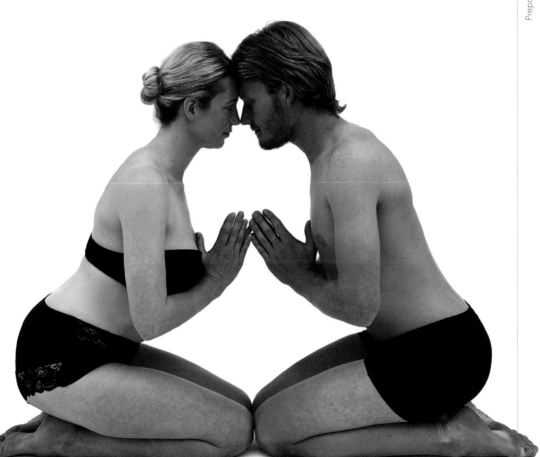

CIRCULATING ENERGY PRACTICE

This is an excellent exercise to start developing your ability to "give" and "receive" energy in a partnership—something that's great for lovers wanting to explore their yin and yang sides, as well as anyone who wants to deepen their connection.

1 *Begin by facing each other, unclothed, between one and two arm's lengths apart. The "yang" partner for this exercise (who doesn't have to be a man) stands with legs together and hands held over his heart, feeling himself to be grounded and solid. Meanwhile, the "yin" partner (who, likewise, needn't be female) stands in a "star" position, legs apart and arms reaching up to draw energy from the skies.*

2 *Reach your hands out so that you are touching each other palm to palm. You'll notice how the energy flow changes: you are no longer reaching up or down, but directing your focus toward your partner. Feel the warmth and life between your hands, and enjoy the sense of connection.*

3 *One of you starts to "send" the energy out into the body of the other, who acts as receiver. After a few minutes, you switch roles. Feel the flow between you and how it changes.*

4 *Finally, try to feel a "circuit" of energy between you. Build energy in your pelvic chakra (see page 38), send it up to your heart chakra, and out through your dominant hand into your partner, who sends it through their pelvic and heart chakra back into your non-dominant hand. (If one of you is left-handed and the other right-handed, you can cross your hands over at this point.)*

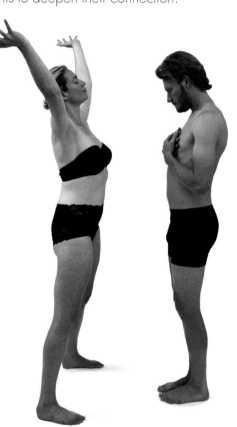

Flow as one

The energy can flow through your chakras and out into your partner, making you a single flowing unit.

Blindfold

This is a good exercise to do in a darkened room, or else blindfolded. If your partner is particularly gorgeous to look at, that can be rather a distraction from the energy flow in your body, so temporarily set aside your sight and just focus on your feelings.

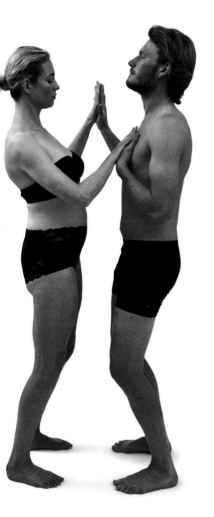

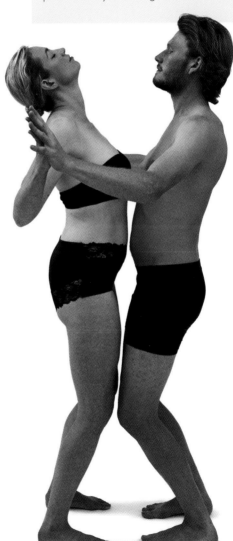

LOVE LETTER EXERCISE

Few things are more traditional, in any culture that uses the written word, than to write a letter to your beloved. This is an exercise that can help communication and reflection within the relationship. When you're alone, begin writing a letter to your beloved. In each stage, write the truth: you won't send the first draft.

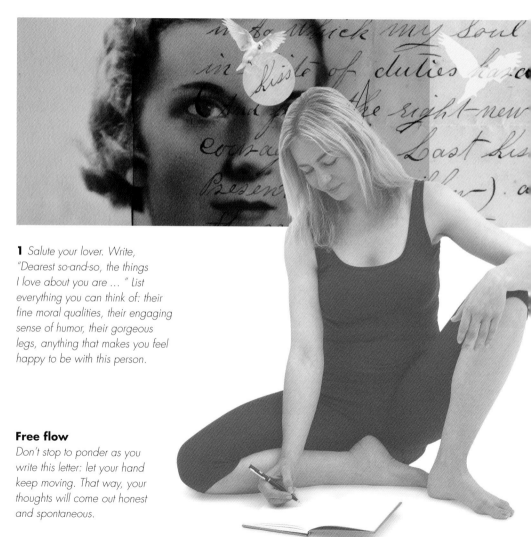

1 *Salute your lover. Write, "Dearest so-and-so, the things I love about you are ... " List everything you can think of: their fine moral qualities, their engaging sense of humor, their gorgeous legs, anything that makes you feel happy to be with this person.*

Free flow

Don't stop to ponder as you write this letter: let your hand keep moving. That way, your thoughts will come out honest and spontaneous.

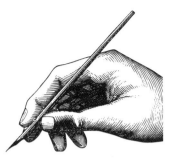

The power of the pen

Most of us are used to typing more than writing, but do this exercise by hand. It helps keep your heart chakra fully involved in the process.

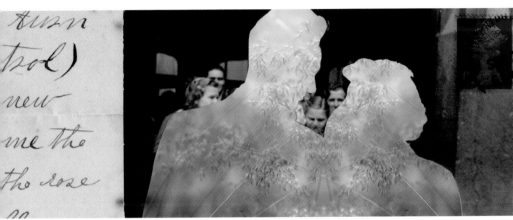

2 *Make your peace. Write, "The times I feel frustrated are when … " Talk about the things they do that bother you, or that you feel are creating any blocks to connection.*

3 *Make your confession. Write, "The times I feel afraid are when … " Admit to your insecurities. Are there things you're worried aren't loveable in you? Are there times when you feel there could be trouble threatening?*

4 *Make your requests. Write, "What I want to ask from you is … " Now you've written down your loves, frustrations, and fears, you should have a clearer picture of what you would like your lover to offer, reassure you about, or do.*

5 *Make your gifts. Write, "What I want to offer you is … " What would you like to give to your lover, from the bottom of your heart? Write it down.*

6 *Finally, rewrite the letter. Leave out steps two and three, just leaving the love, requests, and offers. At that point, you're ready to show it to your lover.*

DRAWING CLOSE

Lovemaking doesn't begin the moment one body penetrates another. The whole point of Tantric sex is that life is one continual blissful moment, and that being true, we need to smooth away our dualistic thinking about what "is" and "isn't" sex. This isn't to diminish penetrative sex, of course; there's plenty of that in a Tantric relationship, if you want it, and it can be wonderful. But sexual energy is just one expression of the energy of the cosmos—which is to say, everything is sex, if we choose to feel it as such. In this chapter, we'll discuss techniques that help you understand your own body and your partner's. Don't assume, though, that this is just "homework." It all brings you closer to bliss, yes, but it's also blissful in itself. These are practices to delight in: they'll make you a better lover through the lovely educational path of pleasure.

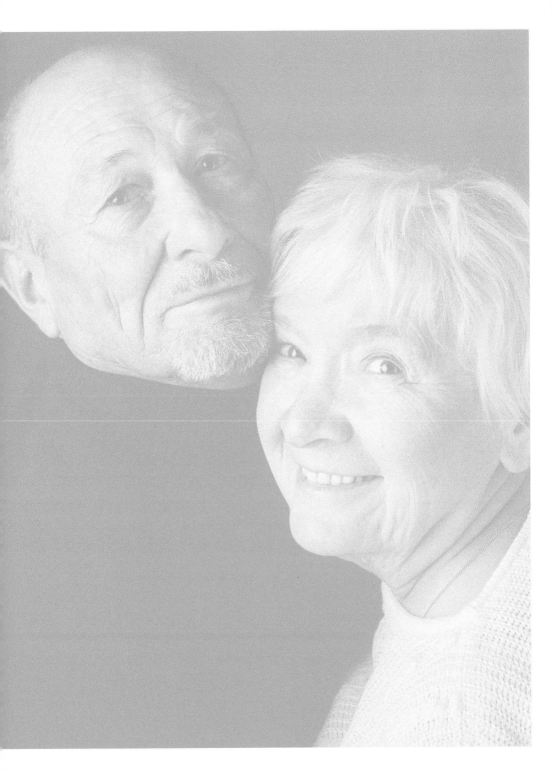

The Many Kinds of Orgasm

F ew things break a meditative state of mind—or an aroused one—faster than the expectation that we "ought" to be having a certain kind of experience. In Tantric sex, this is particularly true for orgasms. We need to be open to pleasure, not prescriptive about it.

There are numerous ways to have an orgasm, and the important thing to understand is that all of them are "right." Let's discuss the commonest:

The clitoral orgasm

Since old Freud informed us that only immature women still enjoyed these, and a fully mature woman should only want orgasms through vaginal sex, this delicious sensation has been maligned. The truth is, many women find it the easiest way to climax, and a good lover honors that.

The G-spot orgasm

Deep inside the vagina (see Understanding the Yoni, pages 172–173) is a sensitive spot—the G-spot—that can, when stimulated, produce a deep, internal orgasm. Some women adore it; others find it too intense. The G-spot is a site for exploration, best touched when a woman is already aroused.

Here's another fact about clitoral and vaginal orgasms, especially vaginal ones: they can lead to ejaculation. Some women release a clear fluid (which is not urine, though many women mistake it for such the first time it happens), that might seep gently or squirt exuberantly.

The penis-based orgasm

Almost every man is familiar with this: semen flows and bliss results. An interesting fact, though: it's actually quite possible for a man to have an orgasm and *not* ejaculate. If he's enjoying himself in a tranquil state, he may have several non-ejaculatory orgasms in a row.

The P-spot orgasm

"P," in this case, stands for "prostate," the sensitive gland near the root of the penis. You can massage it through the perineum, or else internally, with a gloved, lubricated finger gently inserted

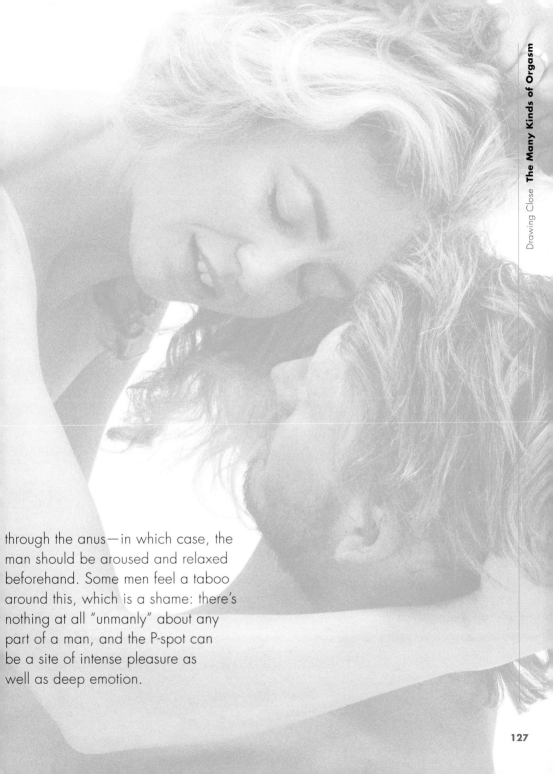

through the anus—in which case, the
man should be aroused and relaxed
beforehand. Some men feel a taboo
around this, which is a shame: there's
nothing at all "unmanly" about any
part of a man, and the P-spot can
be a site of intense pleasure as
well as deep emotion.

127

PREPARING FOR SELF-PLEASURING

Our bodies learn from experience, and your best first teacher is yourself. Self-pleasuring is how we explore our own responses and discover how to enjoy our own sexuality: a good lover knows how to love themselves. This is a good exercise to get yourself in the mood—not just in terms of being ready for arousal, but in terms of feeling strong, proud, and confident about pleasing yourself. You can do it solo or as an enchanting display for your lover; a mixture of both is good, but begin by doing it just for yourself.

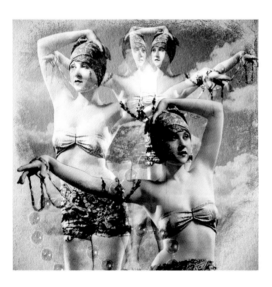

1 *Put on some music: it can be as contemporary as you like. Choose something with a good, solid beat. Start to dance, moving your hips to the rhythm.*

2 *Focusing your energy on your heart chakra (see page 38), shake out your arms and hands. These are the organs that you will be using to pleasure yourself, and they're part of the chakra of love and connection, so wake up their positive energy: you'll be connecting with yourself.*

Physical harmony
Dance is one of the most ancient of all human arts, and many religious traditions embrace it as a sacred ritual.

3 *Focusing your energy on your root chakra and pelvic chakra (see page 38), start thrusting your hips. This is a good way to build up stamina and loosen your back, but more importantly, it's a shameless and open gesture: your body is announcing to itself that you are free to be sexual.*

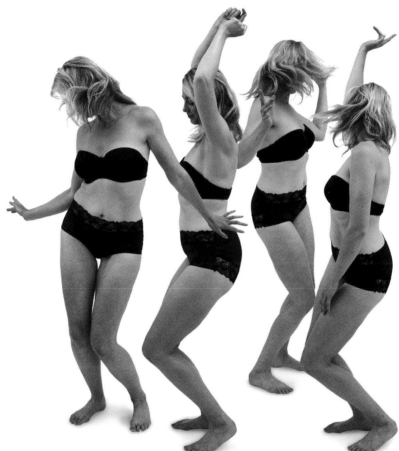

4 *Focus on the sensations in your genitals, perineum, and anus, and swing your hips in a circle. Call it a sacred dance or a burlesque bump and grind; it can be both. Don't worry if you're a little awkward at first: your body will flow freer the more you practice. Feel how your sensitive organs shift and respond. You are making them ready for pleasure.*

Shamelessly happy

Not quite prima ballerina material? It doesn't matter: this is a dance you do for the sensations it wakes in you, not the spectacle you produce for others. Just have fun shaking your excellent booty!

SELF-PLEASURING EXERCISE

Do you worry about having orgasms? Many men feel they tip over the edge too fast; many women fear they can't get there at all, or at least not fast enough to keep up with a male partner. It's time to start letting those anxieties go. One of the key concepts in Tantric sex is the idea of extended pleasure. Put simply, it's a state where we're both aroused and tranquil at the same time. That may seem odd to those of us used to sex where orgasm is the goal and excitement exists only to power us forward, but once you experience that mindset, you'll be in a world of pleasure. It does, however, mean unlearning some habits, so let's begin with a very simple exercise.

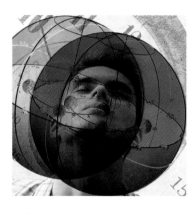

1 *To begin with, prepare yourself by dancing as suggested on the previous page.*

2 *When you feel toned up, confident, and proud of yourself, set a timer to go off in twenty minutes and then lie down in your sacred space (see pages 92–93).*

Relax with yourself

There's no end purpose in this exercise, any more than there is in a breathing meditation. You are simply learning to relax with yourself.

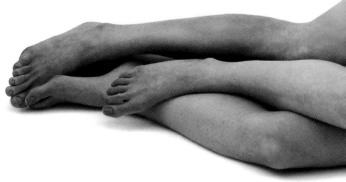

3 *Close your eyes, and begin to touch yourself. Forget your usual rhythm and your usual fantasies. There's nothing wrong with either, but for now, just let your hand explore. Stroke, rub, squeeze, caress: try every kind of touch you can think of, but don't rush yourself. If something feels good, enjoy it.*

4 *The one thing you aren't trying to do is have an orgasm. If you feel yourself close to climaxing, just stop and rest for a moment: run your hands over other parts of your body so that you stay comfortably aroused, then carry on. Don't worry if you do have an accidental orgasm (or succumb to the temptation and go for it): this is an exercise you can do many times.*

Extended pleasure

This exercise can be done by yourself, or lying side by side with a partner, quietly companionable. There is no "goal"; it's a meditation.

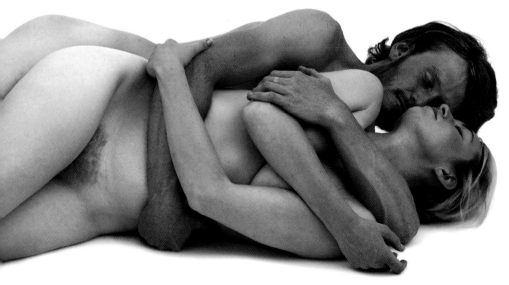

Does Orgasm Drain the Energy?

According to traditional Chinese medicine, which has long been an influence on Tantra, too many orgasms are bad for us—especially if we're male. How do we interpret this in a modern context?

Jing

The theory, according to traditional Chinese medicine, goes like this: our bodies are kept young and vital by an essential substance known as *jing*. Jing keeps us strong, energetic, and fresh, and is the main ingredient in creating yang and semen. Unhealthy living saps our jing, drying us out and making us prematurely old—and too many ejaculations drain us of jing. A man of moderate and healthy habits is advised, therefore, to retain semen as much as possible; there are Qi Gong practices that aim to help a man enjoy sex without losing any jing to ejaculation.

Modern Western medicine would disagree with these claims on a purely anatomical basis: the body manufactures semen throughout a man's life, and as

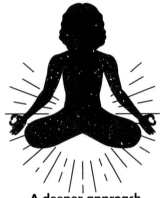

A deeper approach
Hasty sex can sap us spiritually: patience and deep experience are what strengthen our energy.

long as you're in good general health, a doctor would argue you're unlikely to be depleted by ejaculating. On the flip side, you're unlikely to be harmed if you don't ejaculate either, as your body will simply reabsorb the semen. The general rule is that, whether you spend or retain it, your semen won't hurt you.

Modern interpretation

A modern Tantric lover can benefit from interpreting the idea in a broader, more poetic sense. Men are, relative to women, more quickly aroused, quicker to climax, and then subject to a "refractory period" in which their bodies need to rest before they can be aroused again. Racing too quickly toward orgasm may indeed drain the energy from your sexual experience, simply because there are so many subtleties and wonders of spirit and sensation you can experience along the path. Hasty sex is emotionally unsatisfying, and can sap your yang in the spiritual sense: your zest for life and love, and your ability to savor the moment, are virile, vital qualities, and can be better conserved if you take a deeper approach.

CHAKRA MEDITATION

If you've tried sensual meditations on your own, you should be starting to learn how you can draw energy to each part of the body. Now is a good time to start practicing with your partner.

1 *Lie down on a bed next to your lover, with your heads facing in opposite directions. Make yourselves comfortable and, holding hands, breathe mindfully for a few minutes to relax.*

2 *Begin by placing your hands on each other's root chakras—which in this case would be the genitals. Picture a circuit of red light flowing down your arm, into your partner's chakra, back up to their arm, and into you: this light is earthy and potent.*

3 *After a few minutes, move your hands to each other's pelvic chakra, on the lower part of the tummy. Picture a flow of orange light between you; this light is sensual and primal.*

4 *After a few minutes, move your hands to each other's solar plexus chakras, at the base of the rib cage. Picture a flow of yellow light; this light is powerful and confident.*

5 *After a few minutes, place your hands over each other's heart chakras—of course, your hearts. Picture a flow of green light; this light is generous and loving.*

6 *After a few minutes, place your hands over each other's throat chakras. Be very gentle here, as you don't want to impede your lover's breath; just touch the skin lightly. Picture a flow of blue light; this light is clear and focused.*

7 *After a few minutes, touch your fingertips tenderly over each other's third-eye chakras. Picture a flow of purple light; this light is bright and sweet.*

8 *After a few minutes, rest your hands on each other's heads, the site of the crown chakra. Picture a flow of brilliant white light.*

Warming union
Let your energy warm your partner's, and welcome their energy in return.

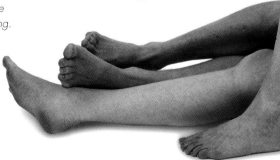

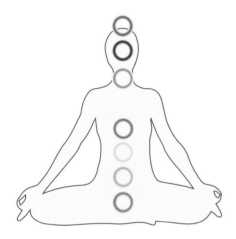

Root to crown

*In this sensual exercise, work up
from the root to crown chakra.*

Intertwined Energies

Should you expect your partner's energy to open
up your chakras? Probably not: they belong to
you, and in the end it's your own actions,
feelings, and spirit that determines how freely
energy will flow through them. However, a warm
and loving interaction with a beloved other is
one of the nicest ways to build up your own
energy, and together you can create a flow that
has its own unique power. Your spirit always
remains your own, but you can intertwine your
energies just as you intertwine your bodies—and
that's a gorgeous form of lovemaking.

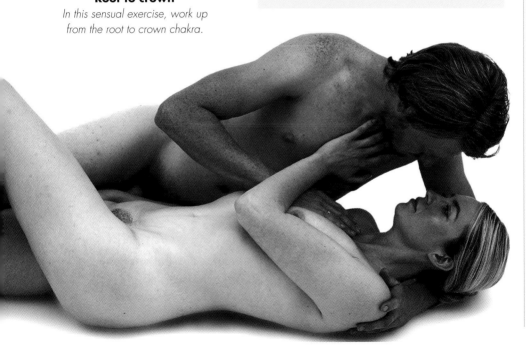

Drawing Up Energy

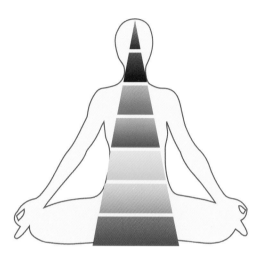

Channel the energy
*Use your focus to draw the
sensual energy deeper and
higher in your body.*

yourself or while your partner is pleasuring you. Remember, there are no mistakes, just a variety of good experiences.

Choose a way of pleasure that you know from experience will reliably bring you to orgasm. Enjoy it, letting the gorgeous sensations build up in you—and be particularly aware of how close you are to climax. Feel the energy building in your root and pelvic chakras.

Slow it down

When you feel yourself getting right up to the edge of orgasm, pause just for a moment. Don't stop the stimulation entirely, but slow it down—and, breathing deeply and calmly, draw the energy up from your root and pelvic chakras and into your solar plexus chakra. Then carry on with the stimulation, your body more deeply charged than before.

Once you're comfortable with this, you can start practicing drawing your energy up to your heart chakra, and perhaps even higher. This practice is one of those things you have to learn by doing, so don't be displeased with yourself if it doesn't work and you either climax or lose your arousal. Enjoy it, and keep trying.

It's time to discuss one of the most important techniques in Tantric sex: drawing up energy before climax. This is the method that allows you to ride a wave of arousal, unhurried and thrilled at once. It takes some practice, so enjoy the learning process.

Having grown familiar with your chakras (see pages 36–39) and gained some practice enjoying pleasure without orgasm (see Self-pleasuring Exercise, pages 130–131), you're ready to try this new practice. You can do it while pleasuring

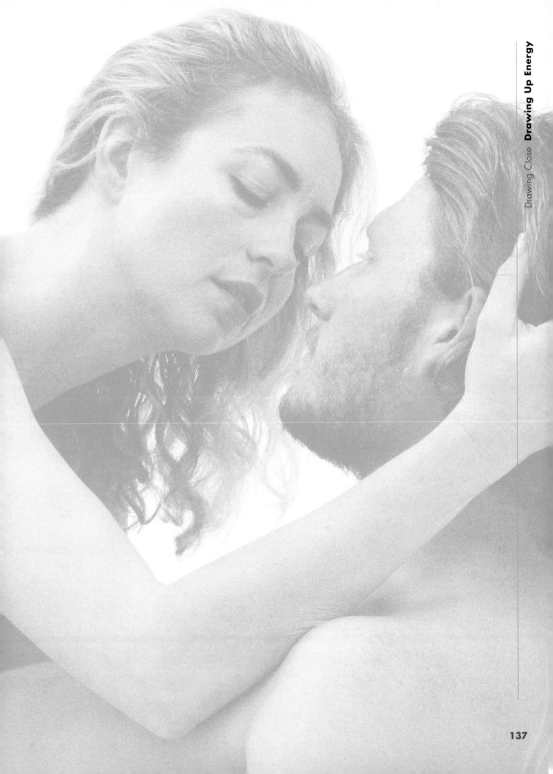

Pressing—Yes or No?

Traditional Tantra, especially Taoism, advises certain physical techniques to delay orgasm in a man. There's a technique known as "pressing" that has been advocated for centuries. The idea is that, when a man gets close to orgasm, he presses with his fingers on a particular spot on his perineum. You can find it with your fingers: feel around for a place that's a little softer than the rest, like the soft spot on a baby's head. Many men argue that pushing on this spot can delay orgasm, and sometimes make it stronger.

Injaculation

There is a medical caveat, though. It can have the effect of causing "retrograde ejaculation" or "injaculation"—that is, semen being released into the bladder rather than outside the body. Now, this is a phenomenon usually experienced as a side effect of certain medications, injuries, or health conditions, but it isn't harmful in itself: the bladder can absorb the semen and won't be damaged by it. However, if it becomes habitual, it can lead to infertility.

A few "pressed" orgasms are unlikely to do you much damage as long as you aren't too rough with yourself. That said,

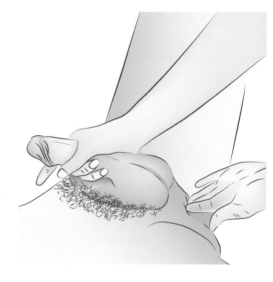

Pressing practice
There are many sensitive spots on the perineum: becoming familiar with them is always good practice.

your body is sacred and should be treated with respect, so we're advising that you keep such methods to a minimum, and work instead on drawing up energy in a non-invasive way (see page 136). If you're very curious, a doctor or urologist is the best person to consult. You can experience a great deal of bliss without this method: exercise caution with your body so you can enjoy wildness and freedom in your lovemaking.

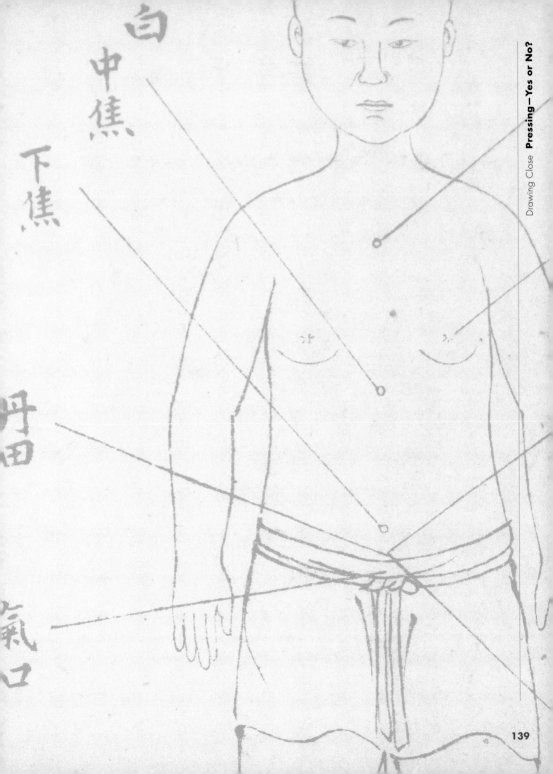

The Hollow Bamboo

As you practice drawing up energy, there's a concept from Tantra that can be extremely helpful. Traditionally called the "Hollow Bamboo," often called the "Inner Flute" in Western Tantra, it's a way of being in your body that complements the understanding of your chakras and Kundalini energy, and can create a subtle harmony of pleasure and peace within you.

What is the Hollow Bamboo?

Picture a channel running right up the center of your body, connecting your energy flow through your sexual organs, adrenal glands, thyroid, and brain. It's the same place we consider the chakras to be located, but rather than seven separate centers, we envision the Hollow Bamboo as an open path which, if not blocked, allows energy—and sexual delight—to flow through the whole body.

The Hollow Bamboo can be impeded by repressed tensions, both physical and emotional. If you're carrying shame or grief inside you, they can act as barriers, the same way that a bit of mud might stick inside a bamboo tube and, should you try to blow down it, force the air to move through a cramped and awkward space.

Release strong emotions

Hence, as you perform the meditations and exercises in this book, it's good to be aware that your feelings may want to make themselves heard. Have troubling things happened to you? Do old memories come up when you try to imagine a clear flow of energy through your blameless body? Keep breathing, relax your muscles, and imagine clean, pure air blowing gently past them. You may find strong emotions released; keep giving yourself that pure air.

When your Hollow Bamboo is open, on the other hand—well, there's a reason that it's also called a Flute: your body can "sing" out a note of sweet, vibrating delight. Hasty or unfeeling sex disconnects our genitals from our hearts and minds; with the Hollow Bamboo flowing freely, all become one, a united self.

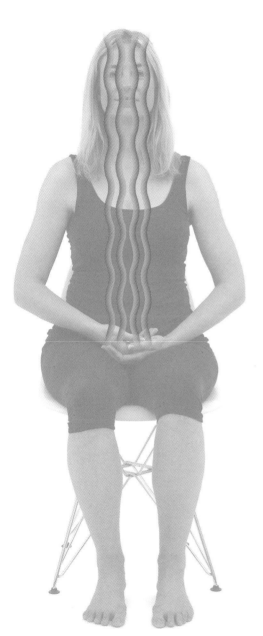

Inner flute

When your spirit is at ease and your body relaxed, energy can flow through you like air through a bamboo flute, sounding a note of pure delight.

Old Wounds

Some people are lucky enough to go through life without serious trauma, but for others, violent memories can stay in the body. Opening up the Hollow Bamboo can, in some cases, create what's known as "relaxation-induced anxiety"—that is, you don't feel open and calm, but stressed, disoriented, or frightened. If this happens to you, try meditating for shorter periods of time; if that doesn't help, it may be your body telling you to find a doctor and discuss whether your old emotional scars need some more help to heal.

Naming Your Beautiful Genitals

For many of us, actually talking about our sexual organs is surprisingly difficult—which isn't good for sex. Think, for instance, of the throat chakra: it is kept open by speaking our own truth. But if we can't find ways to speak freely about what's happening in our root and pelvic chakras, we're hardly going to create harmony within our spiritual bodies.

Choosing a name

Western names for genitals are often either clinical or coarse. Some lovers may actually enjoy the rawness of using four-letter words—and if that sounds like you, then by all means, take pleasure in it. "Rudeness" is a matter of meaning,

not semantics, and if you're speaking to honor the sexiness and power of a sexual organ, then no word you use can be profane. However, you may prefer gentler terms. The traditional ones in Tantra are:
• Lingam, for the penis. In Sanskrit, "Shiva Linga" means "symbol of Shiva"; a common translation is "wand of light."
• Yoni, for the vagina. The Sanskrit word can be translated as "abode" or "source."

These words may appeal to you, but if you aren't accustomed to Sanskrit, you may feel a little strange using such "foreign" sounding words for a part of you so familiar. There are many other Taoist and Tantra terms that you might

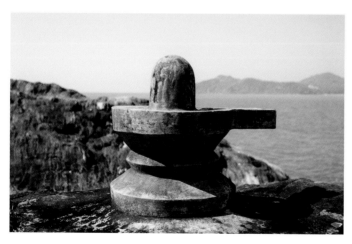

Symbol of Shiva
The lingam meaning sign, symbol, or phallus is an abstract representation of the Hindu deity, Shiva.

enjoy: the penis, for instance, has at different times been called the Jade Stalk and the Heavenly Dragon Stem, while the vagina has been called the Open Lotus Flower or the Jade Pavilion. You could use these names, or make up your own to match your own culture, such as the Diamond Spaceship or Fragrant Rose. You could use these terms reverently or playfully—there's nothing wrong with a little laughter in your sex.

There's no "right" name for these parts of you. The best choice is the one that you and your lover prefer, and that allows your throat chakra to stay relaxed and strong by letting you speak of yourself with confidence and pride.

MALE & FEMALE SELVES

Do you have to be "manly" or "womanly" in order to be sexy? Answer: you have to be human, and there's a lot more to humanity than simple labels. What do you think of when you think of "male" or "female"? Whatever your answer, the truth is this: you have the qualities of both. If you believe you can't be both bold and gentle, tough and nurturing, then you're setting a sad set of

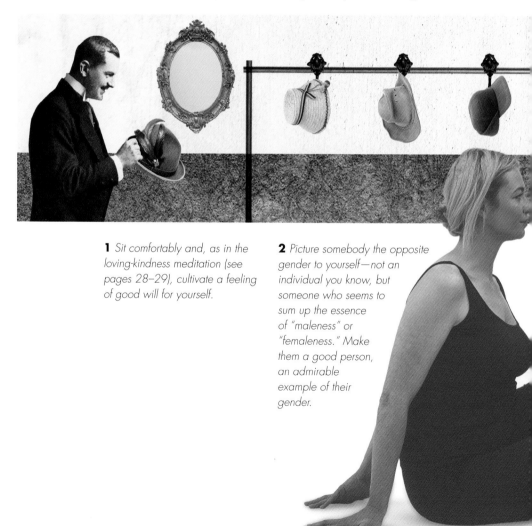

1 *Sit comfortably and, as in the loving-kindness meditation (see pages 28–29), cultivate a feeling of good will for yourself.*

2 *Picture somebody the opposite gender to yourself—not an individual you know, but someone who seems to sum up the essence of "maleness" or "femaleness." Make them a good person, an admirable example of their gender.*

limitations on yourself. And it can hold you back sexually, because if you're afraid of doing something that doesn't fit within those limitations, then you're denying yourself the real freedom your body and spirit need. Seeing yourself as more than a simple gender label isn't degrading yourself: it's honoring just how many good qualities you really have. Try this meditation to set those inhibitions to rest.

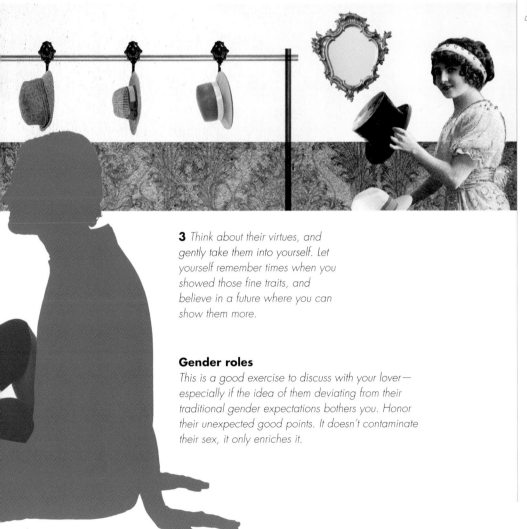

3 *Think about their virtues, and gently take them into yourself. Let yourself remember times when you showed those fine traits, and believe in a future where you can show them more.*

Gender roles

This is a good exercise to discuss with your lover — especially if the idea of them deviating from their traditional gender expectations bothers you. Honor their unexpected good points. It doesn't contaminate their sex, it only enriches it.

SENSORY AWAKENING RITUAL

A gorgeous gift to give your lover is a ritual in which you pleasure each of their senses, one at a time. Sexuality is about so much more than touch: set aside time and enjoy every possible delight. Tantric sex doesn't always have to go on for hours, but this is a ritual you can do slowly, lingeringly, making it a positive holiday. For the person in the "yang" position—that is, the one doing the awakening—this is a challenge to the heart and to the imagination: how many experiences can you make a gift of? For the person in the "yin" position—the one being awakened—this is a ritual of trust, receptivity, and deep, joyful curiosity. In essence, the ritual is simple. Enter your sacred space, and blindfold the receptive lover. Let them lie cozy and calm, while you, the awakener, tantalize their senses with one hidden surprise after another. You can choose whatever you like, but here are some thoughts.

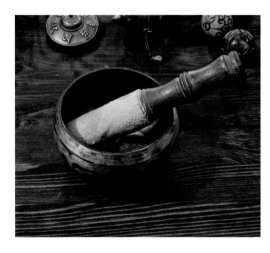

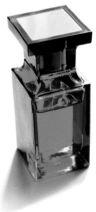

Scent
Essential oils, perfumes, and soaps are your best accessories here. Pass them under your lover's nose, but be careful not to touch their face—not only because some essential oils shouldn't be put directly on the skin, but also because you want to focus on one sense at a time.

Sound
Traditional accoutrements here would be things like ringing prayer bowls and flutes, but be creative. The satisfying snap of bubble-wrap, the "pung" of a struck tennis ball—let even ordinary noises become sensual.

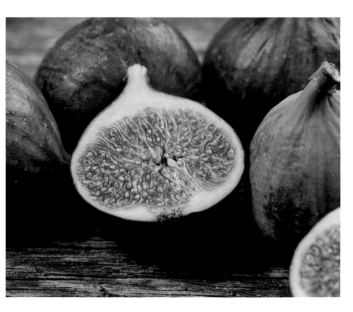

Taste

Choose foods you can give your lover by hand: pieces of fruit, small candies, bite-sized snacks. Go for strong flavors that really contrast with each other.

Touch

Delicate textures like silk and feathers, but don't stop there. Try sensations that push at the edge of comfort—the cold of ice, the prick of a surgical pinwheel, the heat of candle wax (or a wheat pack if you're more cautious).

Be Curious and Open

For the person receiving these sensations, assume a meditative state of mind. Don't feel pressured to endure a sensation that really bothers you, of course, but let yourself be curious and open, as if every sensation were new, and you were, just here and now, discovering what it means to feel.

Watching Your Partner's Climax

Just as we need to understand our own body's responses if we're to immerse ourselves in pleasure, we need to learn our partner's responses—to know them as well as a musician understands their beloved instrument.

Let your lover bring themselves to climax, and watch closely. With mindful attention, study the intimate language of movement and stillness, moans and gasps, loud cries and rapt silence. Nobody responds to orgasm exactly the same way as anyone else, and indeed, different qualities of climax draw different reactions in the same person. This is what a lover needs to see.

Faking it

On this subject, let's address the thorny question of faking orgasm. Women sometimes do this to save their man's pride (and occasionally it happens in other kinds of relationships). If you've done it, hear these words spoken kindly: don't use your body to lie to your lover.

If, on the other hand, you find that your lover has been faking orgasm with you, please understand that, in telling you the truth, she is gifting you with her trust. Keeping her secret was done out of a misplaced desire to make you happy, and breaking it is necessary to give you a deeper kind of happiness. She is pulling out the splinter of miscommunication: it might sting at the time, but after it's gone, you can heal fully.

Whether you are the former faker or her lover, don't blame yourself. There are many reasons why someone might find it hard to climax—at least in the conventional sense (see "emotiongasms," page 54). You are now on a broader and better path, and the pressure is off. Forgive each other and move forward together.

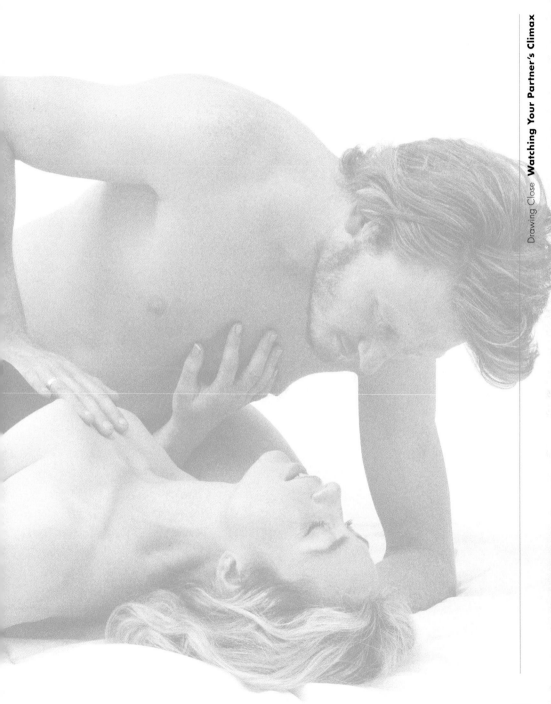

Watching Your Partner Near Climax

So much of the Tantric sexual space depends on pausing and drawing up your energy before the moment of climax. To bring your lover into that blissful space, you need to be able to recognize when they're approaching it.

When making love with your partner (whether through penetrative sex or any other way), be alert for the moments when they're nearing orgasm. It's at those moments that they have the opportunity to draw energy into their higher chakras and carry on to even greater pleasures—and they'll need your sensitivity. It's hard to move climactic energy up the Hollow Bamboo (see pages 140–141) when our lover is busily pleasuring us at maximum stimulation; they need you to know when it's time to ease off just a little.

Observing your lover

You will, of course, have a lot of fun trying it out together, but one of the best ways to begin is by watching your partner pleasure themselves and hover on the edge of climax, much as you practiced in the Self-pleasuring Exercise (see pages 130–131). Your presence can be a warm glow of love and acceptance for them as they work on learning this new skill, and for you, it can be an open-eyed meditation—observing every motion, watching with focus and kindness as your lover shows you, through action, who they are when they are dancing along the edge of orgasm.

As you become more comfortable with each other, you can begin doing this exercise by pleasuring each other. The best way to start is to let your lover lie back and pleasure them with your hands: that frees you up to sit back and watch them hover on the edge of orgasm from a clear vantage point. Later, you can practice pleasuring with your mouth, or by full penetration, but begin by just using your hands and watch as your partner enters their state of bliss.

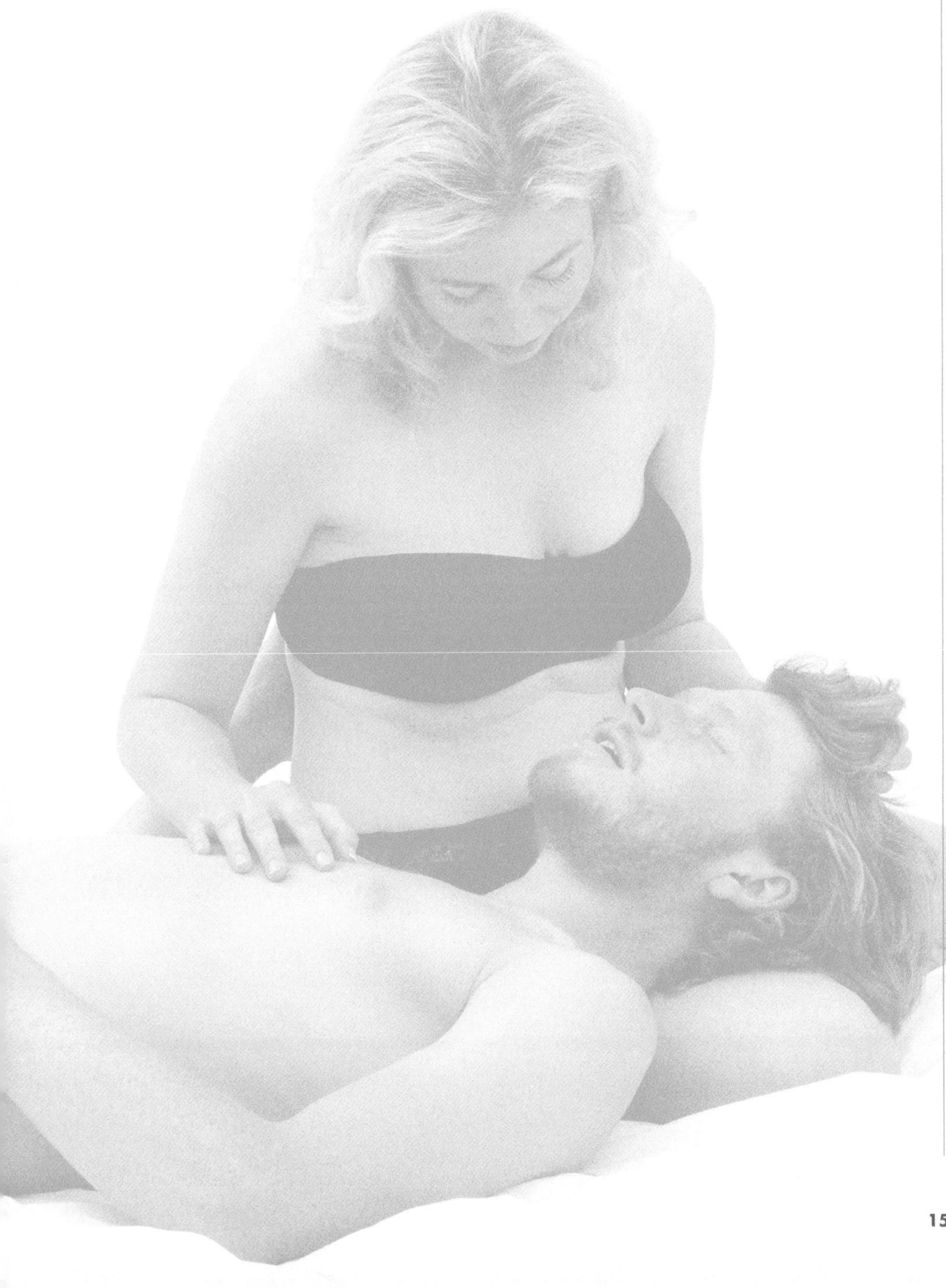

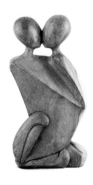

Divine union
*The delicious-sounding name
"Yab-Yum" comes from Tibetan,
and literally means "father-mother."*

THE YAB-YUM POSITION Tantric sex can be done in any position
you like, but one position is a classic within the tradition—not just for intercourse,
but for shared meditation and embraces of all kinds. Practitioners like to say that
the Yab-Yum position symbolizes the divine union of man and woman, Heaven and
Earth. Of course, in modern Tantra this doesn't mean that only heterosexual couples
can do it; if you and your lover are the same gender, you may like to swap around
depending on who's feeling more "yin" and who more "yang" at that moment (see
pages 44–45). It's a lovely position for closeness, intimacy, aligning your chakras,
and sharing the power of your bodies.

Easier Yab-Yum

If you're only just starting to loosen your body
up with exercises, or if you're older or have
any injuries, you may find this variant more
comfortable. The man sits and stretches his legs
out forward, and the woman sits before him and
interlocks her legs with his. Again, you may like
to use cushions to adjust your heights to the
perfect match.

Classic Yab-Yum

*The man or yang partner sits cross-legged—you
can go for a full lotus (feet folded up onto thighs) if
you're particularly limber, but ordinary crossed legs
are fine. The woman or yin partner sits in his lap,
or else slightly raised on a cushion, and wraps her
legs around him.*

Together

When you're finishing a shared meditation or pleasure experience, or warming up to one and discussing how you'll do it, the Yab-Yum is a great position to sit together in.

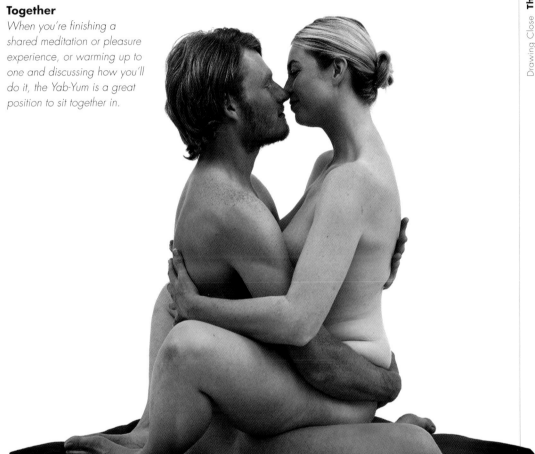

Gazing During Climax

Can you really look your partner in the eye during orgasm? It can be surprisingly difficult—but almost nothing will bring you closer.

Sex can be tremendously uniting, but at the same time, there's an element of isolation to it. After all, nobody can feel your orgasm except you—which means that sometimes, you might almost forget your partner.

Now, that isn't necessarily a problem. Watching a lover "fly" is thrilling in itself, and we needn't feel abandoned by them if they'll fly back into our arms as they come down from the peak, and the essence of sex is, after all, to bring our solitary pleasures into mutual harmony.

Trust

However, Tantric sex means breaking down barriers and letting ourselves really trust, and during the moment of orgasm, that isn't always easy. It's a moment when we are not in full control of ourselves: our bodies have taken us over, and are acting outside our conscious command. To be really *with* someone during that defenseless moment is a step into a deeper relationship.

Gazing exercise

With that in mind, an exercise you should try is this: as you near orgasm, whisper to your partner that you're ready—and then, as you carry on stimulating yourself or being stimulated by them, begin a Gazing Meditation (see pages 98–99). Focus on the darkness of their pupils, the fanned color of their irises, the direct force of their presence.

Some of us may find this easier than others. If you are someone who finds it distracting to focus on the visual because what really excites you is touch or sounds, your lover can help you by giving extra caresses or whispering thrilling things to you. If the vulnerability unnerves you, forgive yourself, but do keep practicing—it's worth the courage.

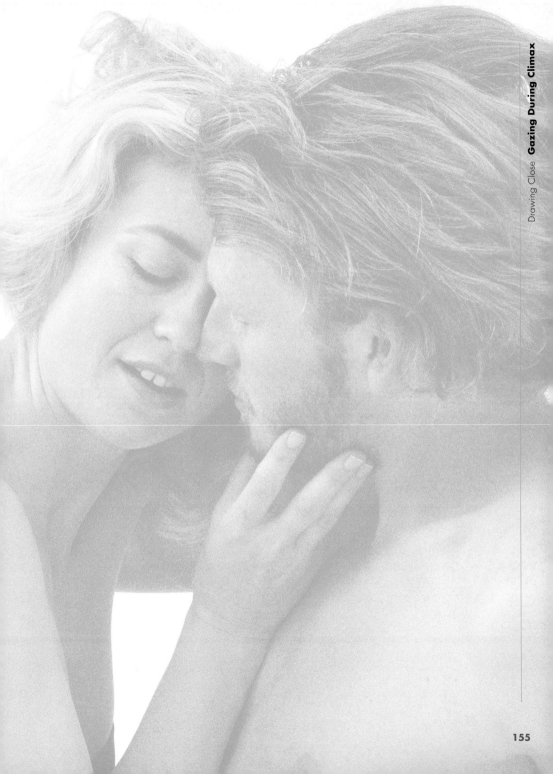

EXPLORING ECSTASIES

Pleasuring your partner wakes up your own body and, if you let it, your own soul. Tantra involves being both excited and relaxed at the same time, and through these giving-and-receiving practices, you can help each other learn this state. Set up your Sacred Sexual Space to be as welcoming as possible as you do these: you are on a journey of sensual discovery. You may also like to begin and end these exercises by doing a bonding meditation such as the Lovers' Greeting or the Hugging Meditation. If they end by tempting you into wilder or more conventional acts of lovemaking, then enjoy them with all your heart—but keep practicing. These are exercises to return to, relax in, and enjoy. By learning to give and receive, by exploring the power of your lover's pleasure and your own, you are diving deep into your sexual journey.

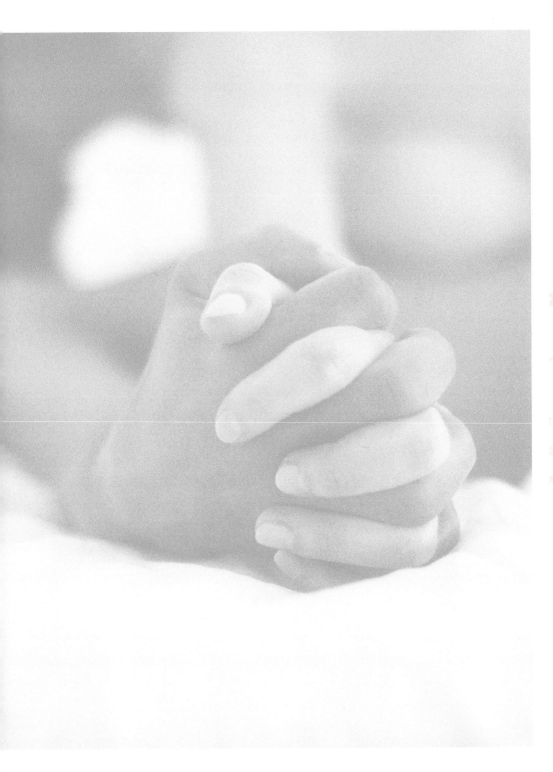

Giving & Receiving

If we ascend to bliss as a couple, does that mean we have to enjoy the same sensations at the same time? Far from it: we can take turns, playing harmonies on each other.

The joy of the moment

There's this idea in many cultures that has caused a lot of heartache for who knows how many lovers: the "true" sexual experience is a simultaneous orgasm, preferably involving penetrative sex. Now, it's not our intention to disparage such moments: they do happen, and they can be gorgeous. What is important is to understand that they're not the ultimate peak of sexual experience—or rather, they don't have to be. A peak sexual experience is simply a moment where you're totally possessed by whatever you are doing, whatever is happening to you.

And that can happen no matter what actual act you're engaged in. Is an orgasm experienced while your lover is generously pleasuring you inferior to an orgasm experienced while you and your lover are mutually pleasuring each other?

Not at all. Come to that, is an orgasm a more meaningful moment of Tantric sex than giving your lover an orgasm? It doesn't have to be: the act of pleasuring someone else can be a passionate meditation that moves and uplifts you even if you aren't especially aroused. Such an experience acts upon your heart chakra more than your root chakra, we might say—but nobody would argue that one chakra is more important than another.

Blissful energy

So: if you're pleasuring your partner, don't tell yourself, "This is sex for him/her; there will be sex for me later." Nor, if you're the one being pleasured, should you tell yourself, "Sex is happening to me, not my lover"—few thoughts can spoil your enjoyment faster. What you are both doing is tapping into the great energy of cosmic bliss—and you are doing that together, no matter what specific act you perform. When it comes to Tantric sex, sometimes you'll want to be swept up in mutual experiences, but you can also give yourself, freely and absolutely, to the experience of giving or receiving pleasure.

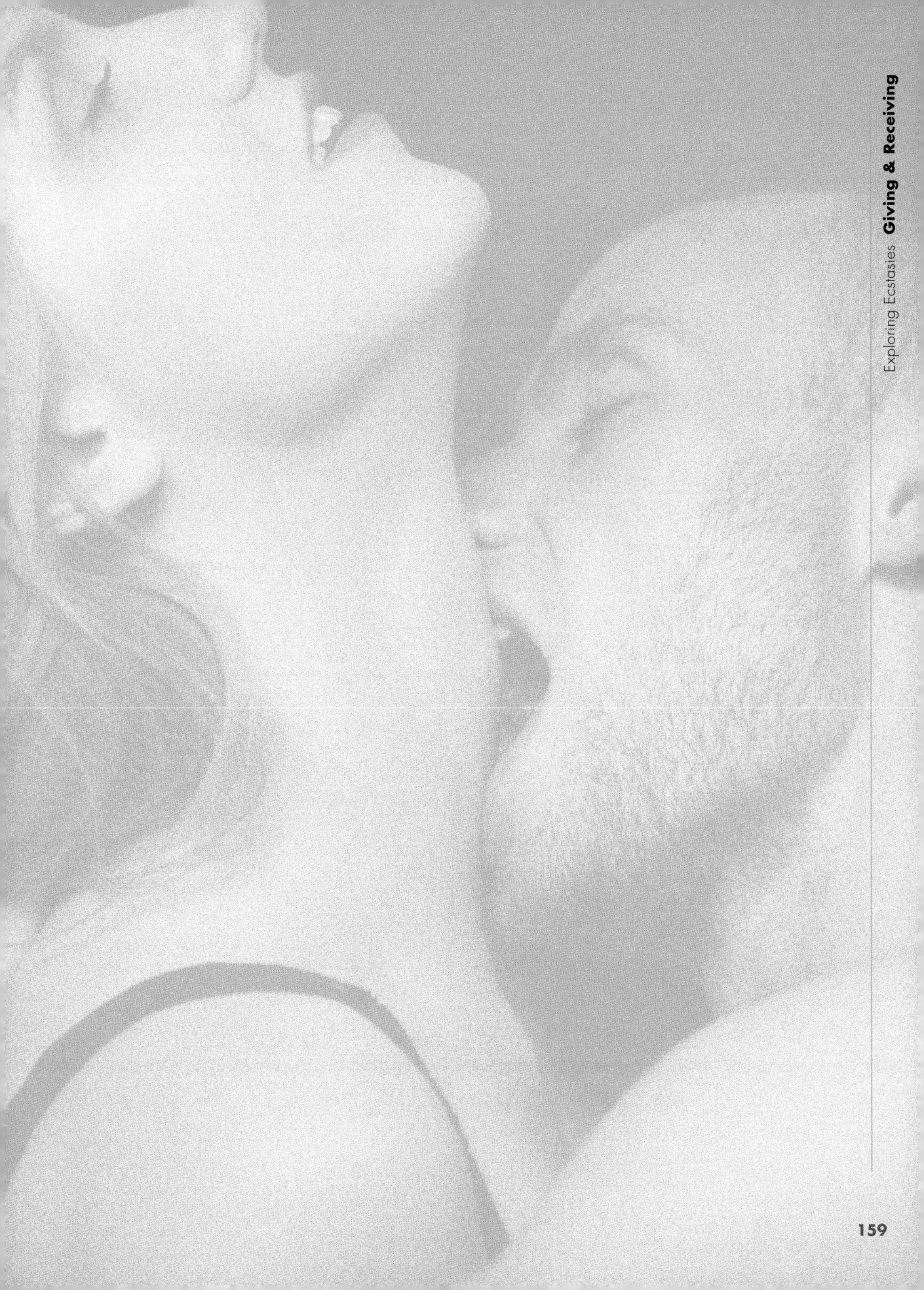

The Power of Touch

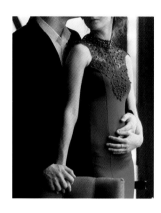

Passionate touch
*Your hand is a sensitive organ:
be alive to the pleasures it can
experience as well as give.*

There's magic in your hands. We are able to use them to shape our world, to speak our thoughts—and touch our beloveds. When you come to caress your partner, you will be using your hands for two purposes.

Receptive
First, your hands will be receptive. Think of how blind people can literally read using just their fingertips on a page of Braille: we can use our hands to "see." There was even a scientific study published in 2014 in the journal *Nature Neuroscience* that suggested that the nerve endings in our fingers can perform some neural processing that was previously thought to be done in the brain itself. Your hands, if you allow yourself be fully aware of them, are a highly sensual organ.

Have you ever stroked a piece of velvet or a soft petal just for the physical pleasure of touching it? This is a pleasure you can bring to your lovemaking. With this in mind, you and your lover will be considerate to each other if you keep your skin and hair clean, smooth, and well-cared for; you can also experiment with oils, creams, and lubricants to make touching a lovely sensation for both of you. If you're giving a massage or a gentle caress, don't neglect your own pleasure. Stroke as if you're pleasuring your own palms and fingertips.

Artistic
Second, your hands are artists. Perhaps you already enjoy the squishy satisfaction of molding clay or the delicate precision of handling a paintbrush—but if you don't, never fear. Your lover's body is your canvas. Psychologists talk about two ways to enjoy life: pleasure and mastery.

By this they mean that there's the straightforward pleasure of doing something you enjoy—but there's also the deep, rich gratification of feeling *good* at something. When we use our hands—the living image of our capacity to act—to draw a shiver of anticipation or a cry of delight from our lover, we are using mastery, not to domineer over our lover, but to paint our strength and skill in pleasure across their flesh.

PREPARING FOR MASSAGE

No matter what part of your lover you're touching, massage can be a ritual. And as with all good rituals, some ceremonial preparation can make it all the better. When getting ready for a massage, spend a few minutes preparing your hands. These are exercises to warm yourself up, both physically and spiritually, before you engage with the body of your partner.

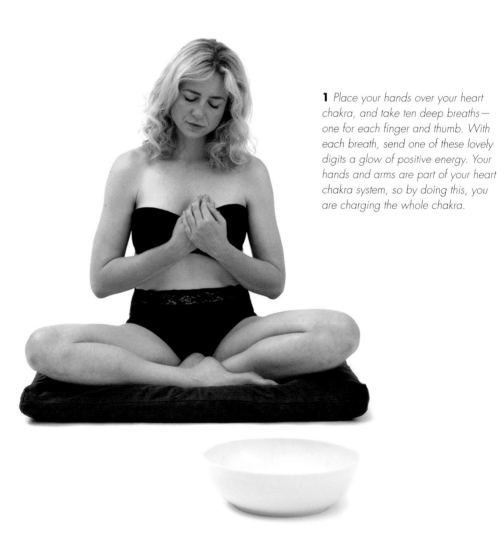

1 *Place your hands over your heart chakra, and take ten deep breaths— one for each finger and thumb. With each breath, send one of these lovely digits a glow of positive energy. Your hands and arms are part of your heart chakra system, so by doing this, you are charging the whole chakra.*

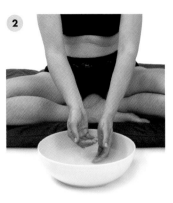

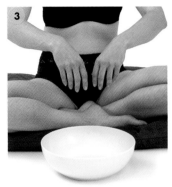

2 Place your hands in a bowl of warm water. It shouldn't be scalding, but enough to relax your muscles and, if your hands tend to be cold, make them more comfortable for your lover. Enjoy the lapping sensation.

3 To dry them, shake vigorously, and keep shaking till they're thoroughly air-cleaned. (Watch out for splashing your partner!) This isn't just to get the water off: the action loosens your joints and releases tensions.

4 Rotate your wrists round and round, letting any knots in your arms or hands ease out. Perform this like a dance move, smiling at your partner, shimmying your shoulders along if you like.

5 "Flick" your fingers outward in a strong, rapid motion. Many modern activities, such as typing, can squeeze our finger joints together, so release all that pressure and send any negative energy flying out of you.

6 You are now ready to begin the massage. End the ritual by repeating the first stage, resting your newly purified hands over your heart chakra.

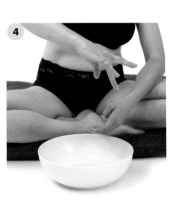

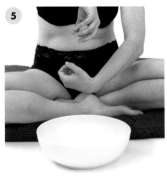

FINGERTIP MASSAGE
Massage can be deep and powerful, but subtlety and delicacy are not to be underrated. In this first exercise, feel out your partner's reactions gently, giving even the smallest points of contact your passionate attention. Before you get into deep massage, you can use your sensitive fingers to test out your partner's skin, muscles, and responses. This exercise is partway between a massage and a caress, so put on music, light candles in your sacred space, and treat it as the lovemaking it is. The important thing about this massage is that you are experimenting with pressure. A lighter touch can be thrilling, a deeper one soothing. Test and try, feeling for the perfect point of contact.

1 *With your lover lying on their front, begin at their feet. Gently touch them, just firm enough not to tickle, and start running your fingertips in a stroking motion, one hand then the other, up their leg.*

2 *Keep stroking up over their behind. Run your fingers up their spine, over their shoulders, touching every part of their back.*

3 *Caress up the nape of the neck, behind their ears, along their jaw. Run your fingers through their hair and over their scalp.*

4 *Let your lover roll over, and begin at their feet again. Caress and stroke all the way up their thighs, stomach, and chest.*

5 *Stroke down their arms and to their hands. The touch of hand against hand is communication, but your lover shouldn't try to reciprocate: let their hands hang loose and just enjoy being touched.*

6 *Finally, run your fingers over their face, gently massaging every feature. End at their lips, and finish with a loving kiss.*

Hair Caress

When it comes to delicate massage, your fingers are not the only option! If you have long hair, it can be a wonderful way to play with sensation: drag it slowly and gently up and down your partner's skin, as if you were painting pleasure on to them. For the caressing partner, your hair can create an enclosed space that screens the outside world from view: breathe in your lover's scent and let there be nothing in your world but them.

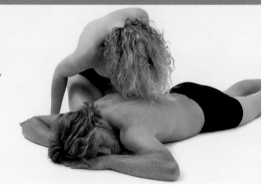

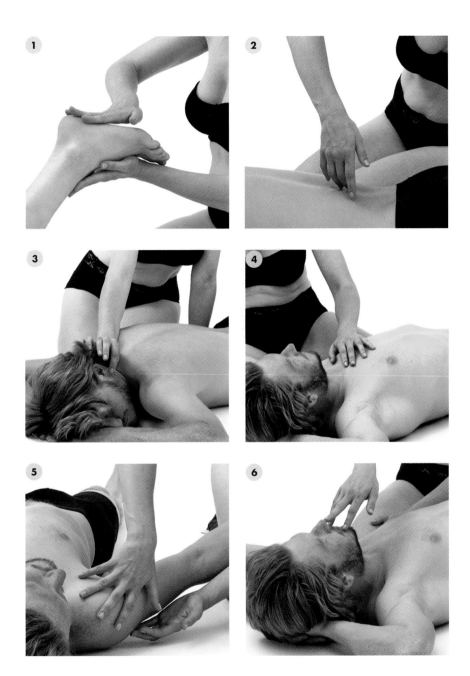

BACK MASSAGE

Modern life gives many of us backache, so this massage is a way to caress your lover's life, soothing away its tensions. It's also an excellent way to begin sensation play. Very few people don't love a back rub. When you massage your lover as part of Tantric sex, though, there's a thought you need to be alive to: the exact level of pressure can be a way to experiment.

The key concept here is what some complementary therapists call "grateful pain." It's part of binary thinking that we tend to believe that pleasure equals good and pain equals bad, but our sensations are more complex than that. Grateful pain is the sore-but-good sensation we feel when someone puts just the right amount of deep pressure on a tense muscle: it hurts, but in a way we want to continue, because it's the pain of a knot coming undone. A massaging lover has to be closely attentive: too much force just hurts and makes us more tense, and different bodies prefer very different levels of pressure. Treat a back massage as a time for the giver to learn how to read their partner's signals, and for the receiver to play with experiencing new and complex feelings.

Sensitivity

Massage can release emotions as well as sensations. Be sensitive to what you're unleashing in your lover. If they show discomfort, go back to a simple, soothing effleurage motion. You are using your strength and skill to melt away the tensions of their world outside your sacred space, so give them all your alertness and compassion.

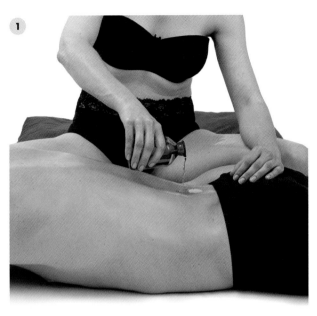

1 Using warmed oil as a lubricant, rub your hands, palms and fingers flat, up your lover's back from hip to shoulder. (Remember, oil destroys latex, so don't mix it with condoms.) This stroking movement is called "effleurage": you use it to warm up and warm down any muscle you're going to massage. Don't use the strength of your arms, but the weight of your body: lean down, letting your natural, physical self be the agent of pressure that sends your lover into a state of relaxation.

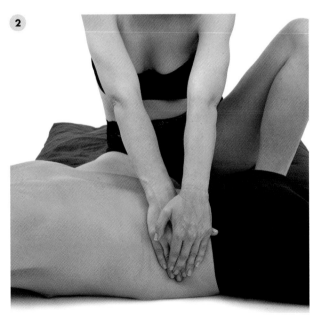

2 Using both hands, one atop the other, massage the area around your lover's hips in a figure-eight, going down around one, up and across, then down around the other. Don't pull them right off the bed, but create a gentle rocking rhythm.

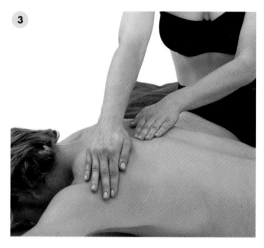

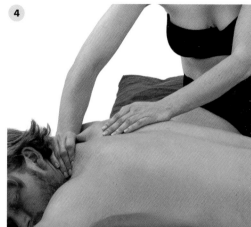

3 Feel along the side of your lover's spine in the area over their rib cage. This is the site of the erector spinae muscles—the strong, flexible supports that hold your lover's body upright. Interlace your fingers to brace them, and rub in circles. A lot of tension can accumulate here, and if you can release it, your lover's body will be freer.

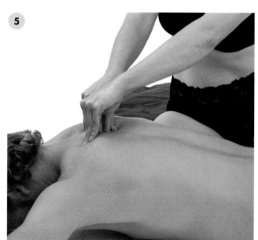

4 Rub around the inside of first one shoulder blade, then the other. There's usually a tight spot between scapula and spine that very much appreciates the right kind of attention.

5 With a scooping motion, squeeze and rub your lover's trapezius muscle—that is, the top of their shoulder blade. This is another area that often feels grateful pain, and because the rib cage is a strong protective structure, you can bear down as hard as your lover can tolerate.

6 When you're done, go back to rubbing an effleurage motion from hip to shoulder.

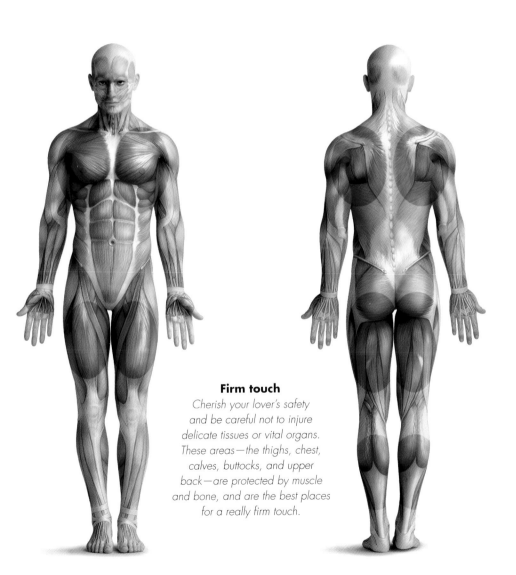

Firm touch

*Cherish your lover's safety
and be careful not to injure
delicate tissues or vital organs.
These areas—the thighs, chest,
calves, buttocks, and upper
back—are protected by muscle
and bone, and are the best places
for a really firm touch.*

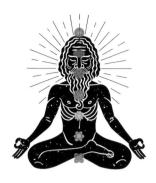

Chakra energy
Everything in the universe is made of energy—and that includes your beautiful body, and your partner's.

CHAKRA TOUCHING MEDITATION Meditations, dances, and exercise can help you become aware of the energy flowing through your chakras, but for Tantric lovemaking, it's also delicious to bring some of your partner's energy into the mix. Warm up your hands (see pages 162–163), and begin:

1 *Place one hand on your lover's heart chakra and the other on their root chakra—that is, between their legs, toward their coccyx. Caress the skin of their root chakra, teasing pleasure into an area that's sensitive both physically and spiritually.*

2 *Gently slide your hands to your lover's pelvic chakra: place one hand on their genitals, and the other on the lower part of their belly. Caress some more. For the partner receiving the touch, this is a good opportunity to practice the state of relaxed arousal that is at the heart of Tantric sex.*

3 *Slide up to your lover's navel chakra; rise and fall with their breath as you stroke. For the receptive partner, draw your energy upward as described in the Drawing Up Energy exercise (see pages 50–51).*

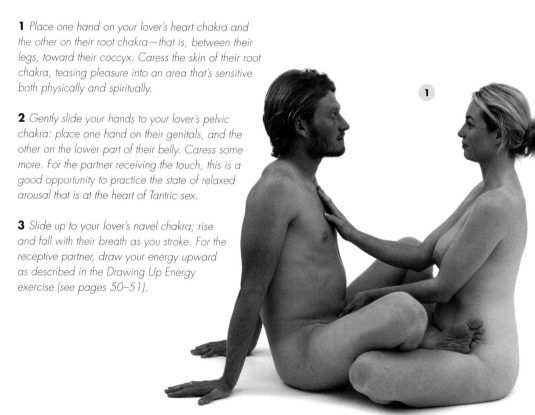

4 *Place your hands over your lover's heart chakra. Slide your hands delicately over their skin—remember, it's chest and arms as well as heart.*

5 *Slide your hands to your partner's throat chakra. This is an act of trust: the partner touching must be very delicate so as not to impede their lover's airways. If you can touch gently and safely, you are cradling your lover's truth: you hold their chakra between your hands while their breath sings free.*

6 *Brush your fingertips over your lover's third-eye chakra. Gaze into each other's eyes and give each other your clearest gaze.*

7 *Finally, run your hands over your lover's scalp for a few seconds, with an upward-flicking motion to draw the pleasure right through them. (But don't snag their hair!)*

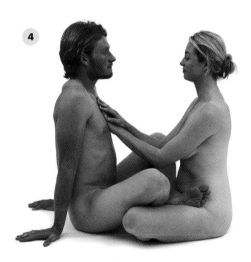

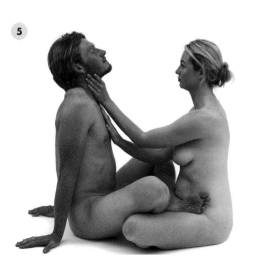

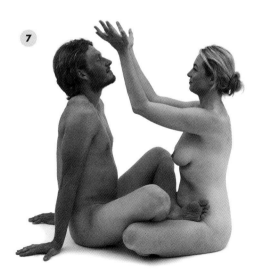

Understanding the Yoni

To pleasure part of our lover, we need to know what we're pleasuring—but the yoni is often shrouded in ignorance. Here are some basic facts to help you be a well-informed Tantric lover.

Love your yoni

Women are often encouraged to be embarrassed about their yonis—which makes about as much sense as a flower being ashamed of its petals. The anatomy of a yoni is subtle and complex, and the better we can appreciate it, the more we can enjoy it.

The clitoris is the only organ on the body that is designed purely for sexual pleasure, and as such it deserves a great deal of respect. However, not everyone is aware of this—it's more than just a little button on the outside. In fact, the

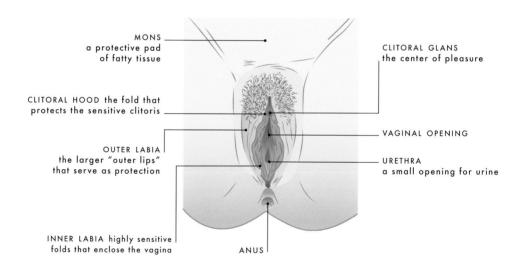

MONS
a protective pad
of fatty tissue

CLITORAL GLANS
the center of pleasure

CLITORAL HOOD the fold that
protects the sensitive clitoris

VAGINAL OPENING

OUTER LABIA
the larger "outer lips"
that serve as protection

URETHRA
a small opening for urine

INNER LABIA highly sensitive
folds that enclose the vagina

ANUS

The yoni
*Everyone's yoni looks slightly different, and has
its own individual preferences on how to be
touched. A wise lover will explore thoroughly
and be sensitive to the response.*

full shape of the clitoris is more like an orchid whose bloom is mostly hidden within the body.

G-spot

Meanwhile, what is the G-spot? There is actually some debate about this still—it could be an internal part of the clitoris experiencing pleasure, but it could also be related to a fascinating organ known as "Skene's gland." This is the site that swells when aroused and can, at orgasm, produce a watery fluid—also known as female ejaculation. Skene's gland, meanwhile, is sometimes called the female prostate, while the clitoris, with its glans and shaft, is effectively a female penis. Gender is not as binary as we think! (See Gender & Love, pages 116–117.)

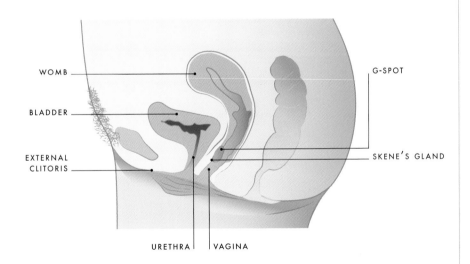

WOMB

BLADDER

EXTERNAL
CLITORIS

URETHRA   VAGINA

G-SPOT

SKENE'S GLAND

The G-spot
Everyone's body is unique: some people love having their G-spot stimulated, others not so much. Embrace whatever reaction feels best to you.

Understanding the Lingam

We have the stereotype that men's genitals are simple—easily understood, easily satisfied. For a really satisfying Tantric love life, though, we should lose that assumption: there's more complexity there than you might think.

There's a good reason why we should stop assuming the penis is a single, uncomplicated organ. We associate bodies and minds: people who are sure that penises are simple entities may find it harder to shake the stereotype that men are simple creatures—sex-obsessed, insensitive, neither capable of nor in need of particular tenderness. Well, that's all wrong, so let's consider the body in a new and thoughtful light.

The sweet spot

When it comes to pleasure, lingams have their sweet spots just as much as yonis do. Exactly where the greatest sexual thrill can be felt varies somewhat from person to person, and a big factor is whether that person has been circumcised. For those who have been, the most sensitive place is likely to be the frenulum—a scientific-sounding name for the soft patch on the underside of the penis, in the "V" shape

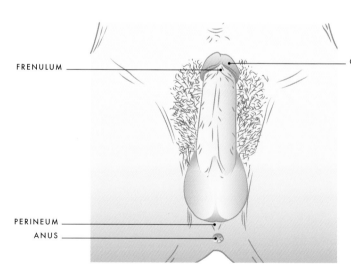

FRENULUM

GLANS

PERINEUM

ANUS

The lingam
The male organ is no more simplistic than the male heart: both need tenderness as well as passion.

just under the glans. The glans can be very sensitive as well, especially in the uncircumcised, and for those who still have a foreskin, there are a great many nerve endings there too. The skin of the penis and testicles can be delirious fun to tease with a light touch. A good lover can have a marvelous time exploring.

Enjoy every part

While we're on the subject, let's talk about the perineum and anus, both of which are full of pleasure receptors. Sadly, it's a zone that many men also feel uncomfortable exploring because of the association with homosexuality—and hence, for some people, unmanliness. Let such fears go: a gay man is just as capable of strength, boldness, nobility, and all the other "masculine" virtues, and we do not attain insight and self-acceptance by rejecting our own bodies. The anus can contain bacteria and is best explored with care for hygiene (latex gloves or a condom over the finger—and remember, oil destroys latex, so water-based lubricants only)—but there's no reason not to enjoy every part of your body, or your lover's.

GENITAL MASSAGE FOR MEN

A genital massage is a marvelous gift to give your lover. Because the penis is often easily satisfied, men can get into habits with their self-pleasuring and forget to explore. This is a way to wake up the body and discover new possibilities. For the person receiving the massage, this is not about orgasm: it's about building up sexual energy and riding the wave. Be responsive and tell your lover how you're feeling—what's good, what you'd like different, and when you need them to ease off a little so you can draw up your energy and hold off climaxing. Breathe evenly and stay as relaxed as you can.

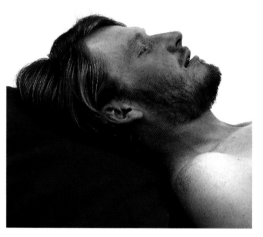

1 *Begin with a fingertip massage around the inner thighs, scrotum, and perineum. This is the area of the root chakra, and should build up a deep, grounded energy. It's so intimate the recipient may feel a little nervous: take deep breaths, and remind yourself that this is the chakra of safety.*

2 *Next, stroke up the shaft. Enclose the head with one hand and draw upward with the other, gathering energy. Use different strokes—soft, hard, straight, or with a twisting motion. Keep the energy awake by changing things up. From here you can experiment.*

The delights of acceptance

In most cultures, men are expected to be aggressive in sexual encounters. That can be fun in a consensual context, but it's great for our emotional and spiritual balance to experience both active and receptive roles.

Giving and Receiving

For the giver, listen and respond. You may also want to observe safe sex by wearing latex gloves and using a water-based lubricant: experiment to find one that's comfortable for both of you. For the recipient, remember: breathe slowly, and don't rush to orgasm.

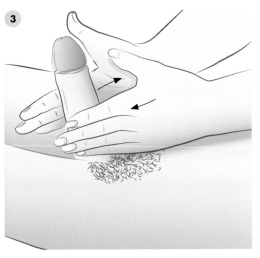

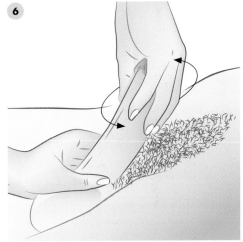

3 *Place your palms either side of the head and massage in a rolling motion. Let your fingers stray to the frenulum and give little brushes, just enough to tease.*

4 *Hold the shaft up with one hand, and with the other, stroke up from the base, across the frenulum, around the glans, and back down again, with an agonizingly sweet feather-tip touch.*

5 *Enclose the base of the shaft with thumb and forefinger, and with the other hand, massage the frenulum with just one finger.*

6 *Stretch back the skin with one hand, and with the other poised above the head and all five digits resting on it, twist your hand in a "juicing" motion.*

177

GENITAL MASSAGE FOR WOMEN

Women often feel rushed during sex with men: their partner's faster pace toward orgasm can put pressure on a lady to get excited as quickly as possible—which is not exciting. A genital massage can help break that stressful association. If you're receiving the massage, remember to tell your lover what you like, breathe, and relax.

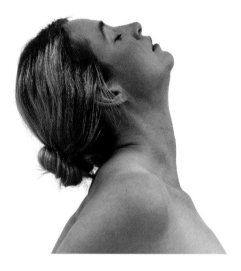

The confidence to receive
Women are frequently expected to be generous, or even selfless—including in the bedroom. Generosity is wonderful, but take this massage as an opportunity to be tended as you deserve.

1 *Begin with a sensual massage warming up the whole pubic area: a feeling of groundedness and safety is important to begin with.*

2 *Next, massage the abdomen with warm, circling motions, whole hand flat on her skin. This embraces her generative organs from the outside, as well as being relaxing: many women are self-conscious about their tummies, so it's important to reassure her through touch that hers is welcome in the sacred space.*

3 *Move your fingers down to the mons, and knead gently. Start massaging her inner and outer labia. (Avoid touching the anus, as transferring bacteria across risks infections.) Stroke up and down, gently tugging, squeezing them together and spreading them apart. Try tapping your fingertips along them as well: the vibration can be delicious.*

Lubrication

As with the massage for men, you may want to observe safe sex here by using latex gloves. If so, it's particularly important to choose a suitable lubricant: women often worry about being too "dry" for sex, and a good lube takes off the pressure. Choose one that's water- or silicone-based so easy to work with.

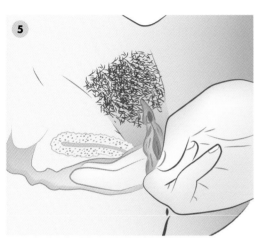

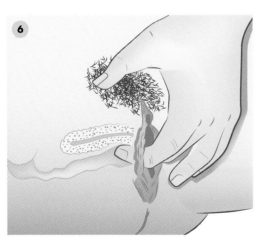

4 *Move to the clitoris: roll it between your fingertips, stroke, tug, and circle around it. Every clitoris has its own preferences, and there's a world to learn about your lover here.*

5 *Slide your fingers inside the vagina—two is a popular number, but experiment to see what feels best for your lover.*

6 *If she's lying on her back and your palm is facing upward, crook your fingers up in a "beckoning" motion until you encounter an area that feels more textured than the surrounding tissue. This is the G-spot, and loves attention. Begin gently, as it can make a woman feel like she has to pee when you first touch it: ease into a pressing and circling massage.*

Body-to-Body Massage

Are your hands the only part of you that can massage your lover? Not at all! Your whole body can be an instrument of caresses. For an exercise of mutual pleasuring that's both deeply sensual and delightfully playful, you can't do better than a body-to-body massage.

Prepare the space

First, some preparation. Ready your sacred space, and lay down some towels on the bed, as this exercise has the messy satisfaction of making a sandcastle or a mud pie. You will need some oil—sweet almond oil is good, being neither too thick nor too thin, or you can buy scented commercial oils that smell lovely. Remember that such things destroy latex, so don't mix this exercise with anything that would need a condom: consider it an end itself rather than "foreplay"—or, if you do end up wanting penetrative sex, be prepared to preface it with a warm, shared shower or bath.

Next, slather each other in oil, enjoying every inch of your partner's skin. The nicest way is to put a scoop in your hand first and stir it with your fingertips so it warms up: that way, you can start with a sigh rather than a shiver! Note: if you're on the handsomely hairy side, use more oil to make sure nothing snags.

Play freely

One of you should lie down on the towels, and the other positions over them. Take some weight on your hands and knees (or hands and feet if you're feeling limber enough to massage them with your back rather than your front), and start gliding up and down against them. With the changing fit and pressure of bodies on the move, your every bulge and bump is a massage tool. Take turns to be the reclining and the rubbing partner, and slide together every way you can think of. This is free play, so there are no formal moves—just the slippy, squishy, slithery pleasure of flesh on flesh.

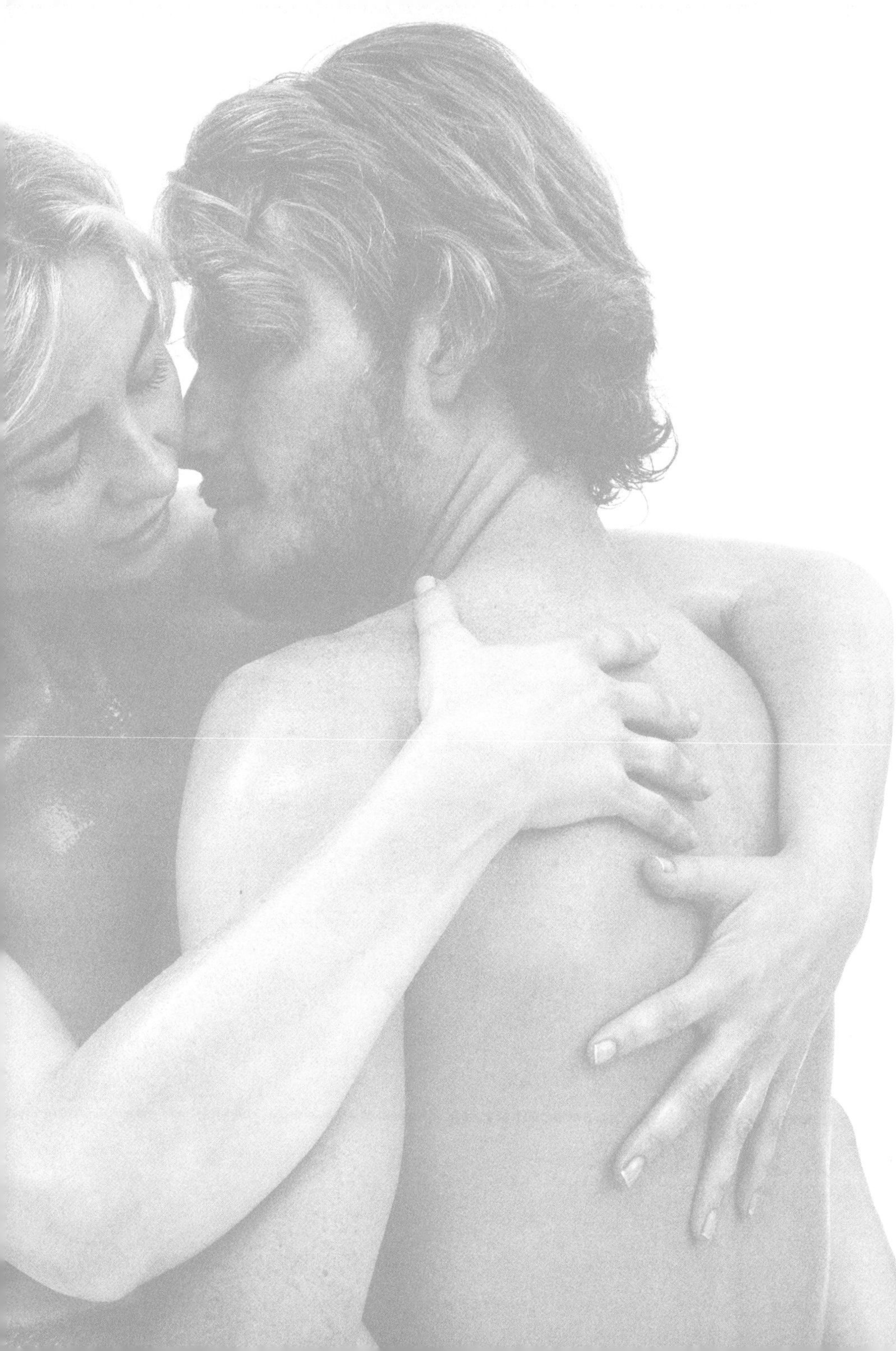

Sex & Stillness

I n Tantric sex, we talk a lot about a state of mind that's both aroused and relaxed, but for the inexperienced, that can sound confusing. Here's a lovely exercise that can help you get comfortable with it.

In non-Tantric sex, there's often a lot of anxiety about "performance." Well, time to lose those expectations. Whatever happens during Tantric sex *is* Tantric sex—there is no "failure" or "problem" as long as we're full of cosmic bliss and open acceptance.

Enjoy your arousal

So, for this exercise, approach it as a meditation. Take your time over it: it's a practice for late at night when you feel ready to drift off together, or for a lazy weekend morning when there's nothing to do but lie in bed and enjoy each other's company.

Begin with a Chakra Touching Meditation (see pages 170–171) to draw close, and then caress, massage, kiss, and enjoy each other until you feel ready to make love.

Choose a position in which you can be comfortable for a long time. Lying down with either partner on top is good, especially if the riding partner is happy taking some weight on their legs and arms. If your genitals are at the right angle for each other, though, the best of all may be spooning: the "inner spoon"

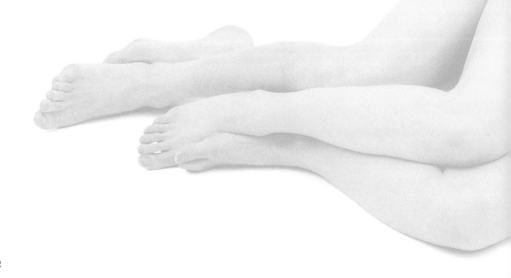

should set up a pillow at whatever point on the bed she wants to rest her head—which may be near her partner's, or may be at a steeper angle to him. You'll enjoy having as much skin-to-skin contact as possible, but if your torsos aren't close, you can always wrap your legs around each other.

Focus on the connection

Next, go into penetrative sex—but however tempting, don't thrust. Just lie together, interlocked. Really focus on the sensations you're feeling at the place where you're joined; perhaps squeeze and flex to send each other little greetings. The man's erection may wax and wane, but remember, that doesn't matter. If you slip apart, either start again or move to a simpler embrace. Let yourselves experience simple penetration with no rush: safe, calm, and together.

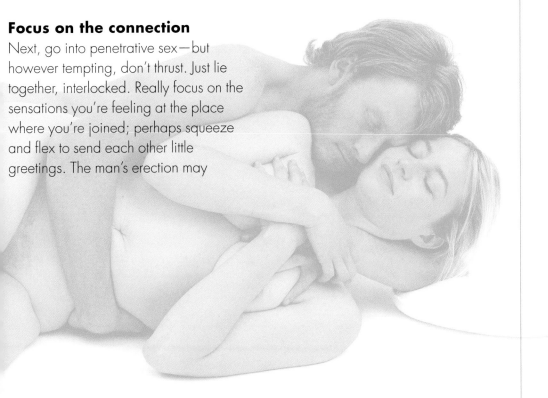

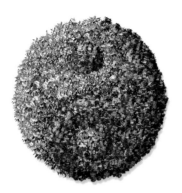

Embody yin and yang
You can embody the yin and yang while pleasuring each other.

THE YIN–YANG 69 MEDITATION
Want to share mutual pleasure and meditate at the same time? This is a sensual exercise that allows you to spin out your arousal in tranquil harmony. You may have heard it called the "sixty-nine" position—but have you ever noticed that when you and your partner lie together using your mouths to pleasure each other's genitals, you also form an image of the yin and yang? You can use that icon to help you embody the quality of mutuality.

1 *Lie down naked with your partner, top to tail, and bring your mouths close to each other's genitals. Don't start orally pleasuring them: you may like to do this when you've finished the meditation, but for now, just rest your lips against their sensitive parts and let your breath be the sole stimulation.*

2 *As you breathe energy into your partner and enjoy the energy they are breathing into you, close your eyes and feel yourself as you are: both yin and yang. You may recall that each fish-shape of the yin-yang icon has a circle of its opposite right at the center of it. Where is it with you in this position? In your head: your third-eye chakra, the chakra of insight.*

3 *Fill your mind with purple light, the color of the third-eye chakra, and continue to breathe. If you are the "yin" partner, let your body tingle with responsive pleasure and focus on the active exhalation; if you are the "yang" partner, feel your body flowing with strength and focus on the receptive inhalation.*

4 *You can conclude this meditation with pleasuring each other more directly. If you do, begin slowly: tease each other with your tongue-tips and prolong the calm excitement as long as you can.*

Mutuality

Male or female, dominant or submissive, giving or receiving, nobody is entirely yin or yang. You can choose to immerse yourself in a state of yin or a state of yang for a while, but your full spirit is always going to be more subtly intermingled. What nicer way to meditate on this truth than while enjoying some lovemaking?

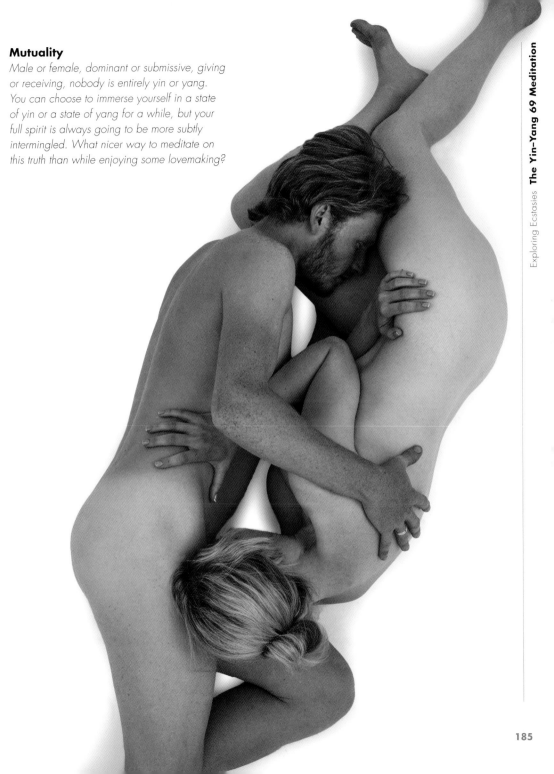

Fantasies & Freedom

With all this talk of mindfulness and awareness, where do sexual fantasies fit in the picture? The answer is that they're an excellent way to learn about ourselves: we just need to keep them in balance, so that they enrich our love lives rather than distracting us from them.

Be present with your lover

When it comes to self-pleasuring, you may simply need fantasies to keep you going. You should certainly try self-pleasuring without fantasies so you can focus meditatively on your own sensations, but there's no need to eliminate them from your repertoire entirely. You are, after all, not getting much input from anyone else, so you may have to become your own lover.

With a partner, it's a little more complicated. Imagination is central to sex, but to rise together, you need to be *together*. For that, you have to be present with your lover: fantasies that take you away from them can drain the emotional energy out of the room. Again, if they're pleasuring you and you're being entirely receptive, then that may be perfectly fine, but some sex is more mutual.

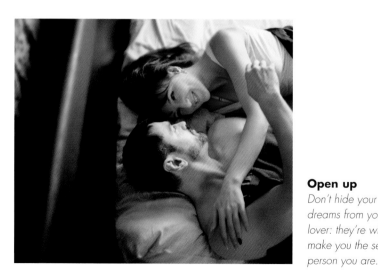

Open up
Don't hide your secret dreams from your lover: they're what make you the sexy person you are.

Share your fantasies

Consider this: what is it about your fantasies that excites you? If you can identify that, then you can use them to become more present with your partner: you simply need to incorporate that element into your lovemaking. Do you love to picture a beautiful bottom or a man in uniform? Your lover can give you that. Is there a certain dynamic that always thrills you—swept-off-your-feet, grandly in control, meekly submissive, wildly romantic? Create that dynamic in your Sacred Space (see pages 92–93).

This is, of course, easiest if you and your partner's fantasies are exactly compatible, but if there's only moderate overlap—well, that's what giving and receiving are for.

Use the Tantric space to create acceptance and safety. Be honest with yourself and your lover about what really turns you on. Your sexual self is what it is, and if you deny it, it'll only become a barrier. Bring it into your sacred space and let it out to play.

DEEP IN PLEASURE

There is nothing quite like the touch of one body inside another. Some manuals give dozens, or even hundreds, of sexual positions to try, many with poetic names—and many very similar to one another, only with a slight change in the angle of a leg or arm. We won't do that here, because the truth is that you and your partner will discover, in an intimate body-to-body conversation, exactly what feels right for you. Different kinds of sensation play, different thrusting patterns, different partner dynamics—these are the stuff of experimentation, of bringing your whole attention to bear on the delicious sensations of your body. The best sex is the sex that makes you happy, body and soul—and what kind of sex that is will change from day to day, moment to moment. It's all yours to discover.

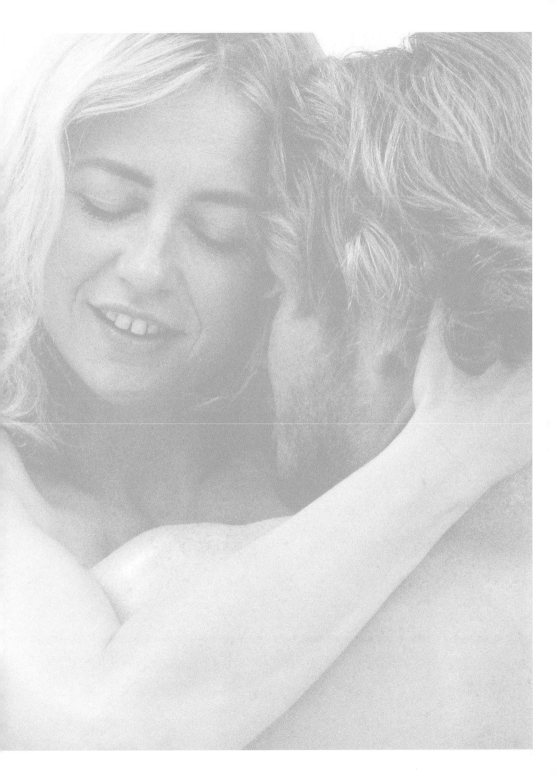

EMBODYING YIN & YANG

Whether you're male or female, yin and yang is within you. You can play with both to enrich your love life. We know that ancient wisdoms tend to come out of times that were, let's agree, not exactly feminist. How do we balance the modern understanding that equality is right—indeed, morally necessary—against the idea that "yin" is female and "yang" is male? If you're a same-sex couple, in a way things are easier for you: you know that you are both equally yin and yang, and can make love according to the needs of your spirit in the moment. But for an opposite-sex couple, the same can be true. The best solution is to play with the idea. Men contain elements of yin and women of yang, and a lively relationship can enjoy many combinations.

To be a "yang" partner

Yang is active, creative, forceful. If you want to make love in a state of yang, you are bringing energy and wildness into the sacred space, an untamed spark of pure life. A yang partner plays the "dominant" role, but remember: dominant, not domineering. Yang is as much about skill and creativity as it is about strength, and a good yang partner takes responsibility for their lover's safety and pleasure, being both masterly and worthy of trust.

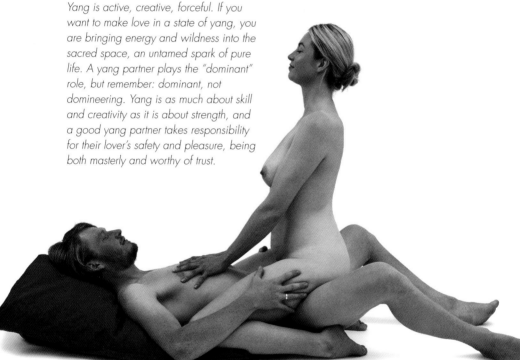

Combine Roles

Whatever your gender, you can delight in both roles—or, indeed, you can decide to make yourself a combination of both, just as the yin–yang symbol shows the two elements entwined. You are part of the universe, and as such, infinitely intermixed, and capable of any pleasure you choose.

To be a "yin" partner

Yin is receptive, transformative, mystical. If you want to make love in a state of yin, you are offering your partner devotion and passion. It's somewhat analogous to what modern sexual experimenters call a "submissive" state—but please note, this does not mean "inferior." Devotion and submission are a gift offered to a lover from a state of empowerment: you bestow yourself, for as long as you choose to bestow yourself, because you are a prize beyond riches.

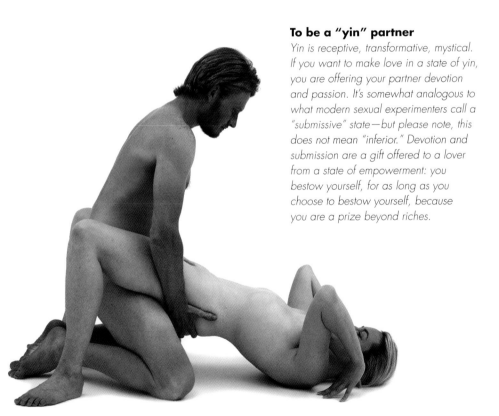

191

YANG-DOMINANT POSITIONS
If you and your lover want to go wild with a male "yang" partner taking the lead, these positions make it easy for you. Gather your energies and prepare for passion.

Behind the Lady

Kneeling, bending, or crouching, the woman positions herself to be entered from behind. This is a position for deep thrusting that often touches the G-spot; it also places little strain on the man and can be sustained for a long time—though the woman may benefit from being propped up on some cushions if her arms get tired. A generous man may also like to reach round to her clitoris.

Lying down, man on top
A classic position, in which the woman can open and embrace her lover while he's free to thrust. He may reach orgasm quickly in this pose, so be prepared to stop and rest at intervals (or change positions to give his arms a rest).

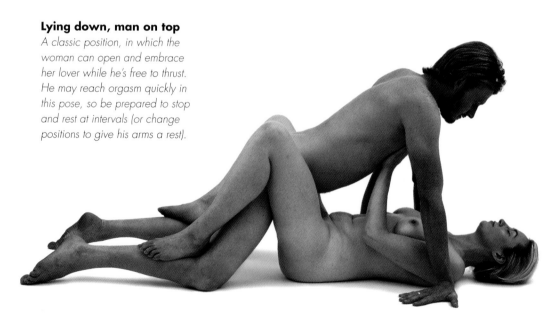

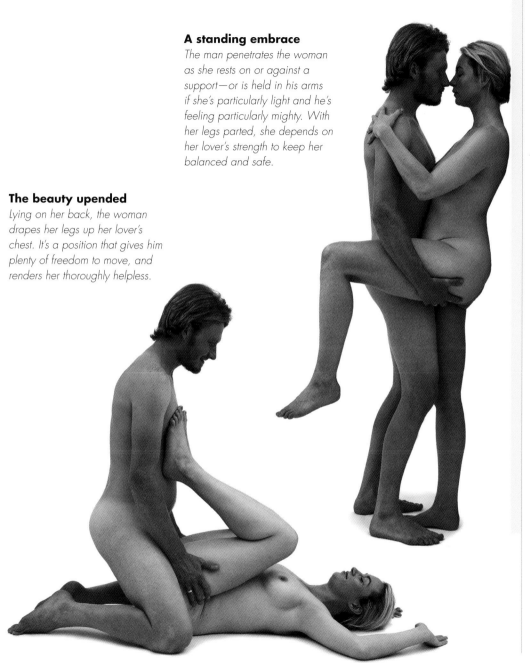

A standing embrace

The man penetrates the woman as she rests on or against a support—or is held in his arms if she's particularly light and he's feeling particularly mighty. With her legs parted, she depends on her lover's strength to keep her balanced and safe.

The beauty upended

Lying on her back, the woman drapes her legs up her lover's chest. It's a position that gives him plenty of freedom to move, and renders her thoroughly helpless.

YIN-DOMINANT POSITIONS "Yin" may sometimes suit a

submissive role, whether played by a man or a woman. That said, there's another possibility: a lady who wants to embody yin—but who chooses to take the lead role.

The reversed ride

This is a position that works delightfully for some lovers and not so well for others, depending on the relative angles of their genitals. If you fit right, it's a powerful position for the woman and a gorgeous view for the man—besides giving him easy access to fondle her bottom.

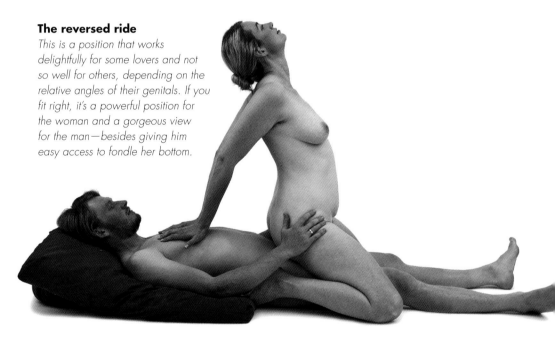

The straddled thigh

With some delicious wiggling into place, the woman can find a position that allows her to grind her clitoris against her lover as well as enjoying the penetration.

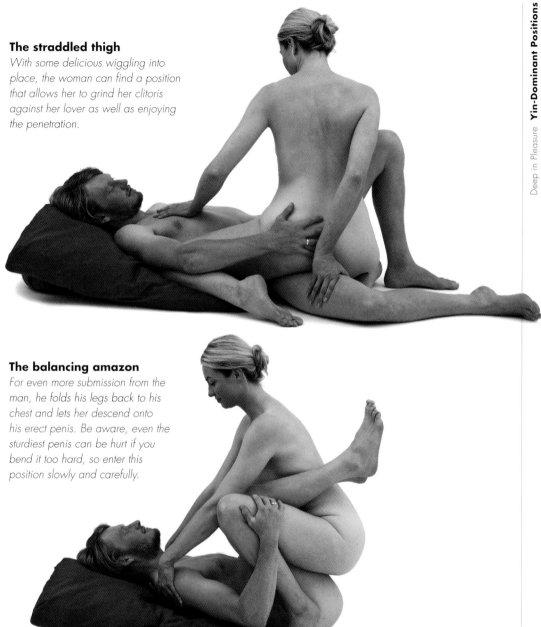

The balancing amazon

For even more submission from the man, he folds his legs back to his chest and lets her descend onto his erect penis. Be aware, even the sturdiest penis can be hurt if you bend it too hard, so enter this position slowly and carefully.

YIN & YANG BALANCED POSITIONS
Sometimes what you want most is to meet each other as equals in passion and power. For those moments, these are positions of mutual equality.

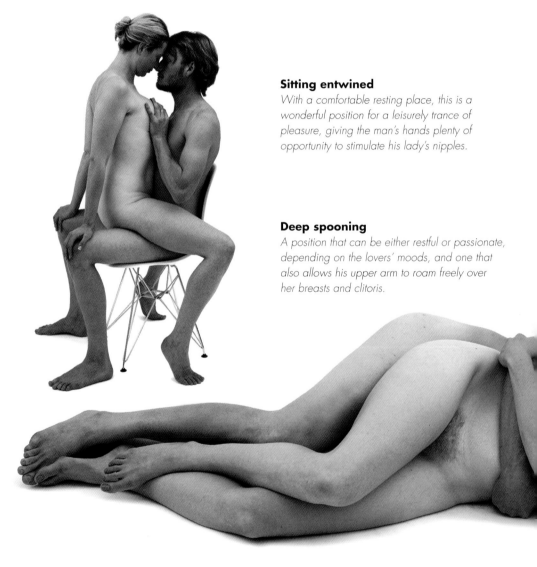

Sitting entwined
With a comfortable resting place, this is a wonderful position for a leisurely trance of pleasure, giving the man's hands plenty of opportunity to stimulate his lady's nipples.

Deep spooning
A position that can be either restful or passionate, depending on the lovers' moods, and one that also allows his upper arm to roam freely over her breasts and clitoris.

The Yab-Yum

You can read more about this on pages 152–153, but it's a classic for a reason: it allows you to merge together face to face.

A lover's hug

This is one to roll around in and change as often as you need to in order to keep your legs comfortable. It's also one of the most natural and tender positions you can try.

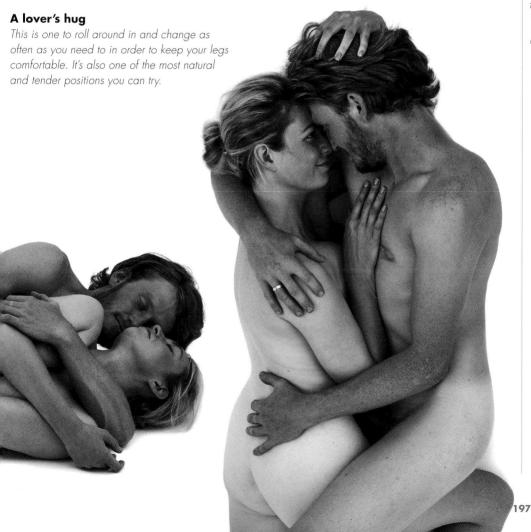

The Power of Tension

Want to conserve your energy during lovemaking? Your muscles have more power than you might think: if you tense them in particular ways and combine those ways with some breathing exercises, the effects could surprise you.

Many men feel the honorable desire to delay their orgasms in order to carry on making love to their partner. Of course, just because you have an orgasm doesn't mean you have to stop making love: Tantric sex rests on the idea that there's far more to lovemaking than penetration, and much of it doesn't depend on an erect penis.

However, an orgasm can disrupt the flow of the moment, so it's quite understandable that sometimes, a man feels the need to stop himself. The methods some men use, though, can be downright discouraging—from trying to think of something very boring, which separates you from the lovemaking moment, to thinking of something disgusting, which is hardly a sensual pleasure! Gentlemen: do not do this to yourselves. There are better ways.

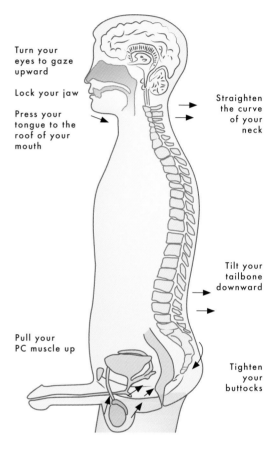

Turn your eyes to gaze upward

Lock your jaw

Press your tongue to the roof of your mouth

Straighten the curve of your neck

Tilt your tailbone downward

Pull your PC muscle up

Tighten your buttocks

Squeeze your anus tight

Body lock
To lock your body and delay orgasm make nine rapid contractions as shown here.

Locking the Gate

This is a traditional technique known as Locking the Gate. When you're inside your beloved and feel climax approach, and you're so excited that you really don't have time to redirect your energies up your Hollow Bamboo (see pages 140–141), try this instead: make nine rapid contractions to tighten up your body as shown in the diagram. With each flex, draw a deep breath right down to the base of your abdomen and hold it there until you release the clench. You are, in effect, "locking" the orgasmic power back into your body—which allows you to keep making sweet love to your dear one.

When you have done this, let your breath gently exhale. Start to relax your body: begin by letting go your neck, head, and back. Let down the pressure in your PC muscles more slowly, making sure that your orgasm has been, for the moment, stopped in its tracks. (If not, keep repeating the clenches in sequences of nine.)

Then relax completely into the arms of your beloved, who should give you plenty of affection for your excellent efforts.

Can We Be Naughty?

Tantric sex is supposed to be spiritual —so that means it has to be pure and virtuous, right? Wrong. If your tastes run to the kinkier side, Tantra can be great for you too.

Tantra is a noble tradition, but it's not a respectable one. It was never meant to be: it was a creative, primal, convention-breaking spiritual school. Sensation play can be a great way to explore, so let's discuss a few toys you might incorporate into your play:

Vibrators and dildos

What's the difference? Dildos are simply phalluses, while vibrators, well, vibrate. The latter might be phallus-shaped, but you can also get shapes to pleasure the clitoris, to attach to a ring around the penis, to reach inside for the G-spot, or even to imitate the action of a tongue. It's good to shop from a place where you can try before you buy—try on your hand, of course, not your genitals. The main distinction in sensation to look out for is that some create a finer, more "stingy" vibration, while some create a deeper, more "rumbling" sensation. Experiment to see what you like.

Impact toy

There's nothing new about adding some playful swats into your sex; the Kama Sutra has a whole section on love-blows. You can use many objects, but the commonest are:

Floggers

That is, whips with many flat tails. The softest are made of fur; medium-soft are made of suede; the sharpest are leather or rubber.

Single-lash whips

A more extreme sensation, and requiring more skill in the wielder.

Crops and canes

Very painful, though sometimes in a delicious way.

Paddles and straps

Producing a wide stripe of sensation—be careful not to cause bruising or broken blood vessels.

The main distinction is between "stingy" and "thuddy" sensations. Anyone using these needs to be very respectful of their

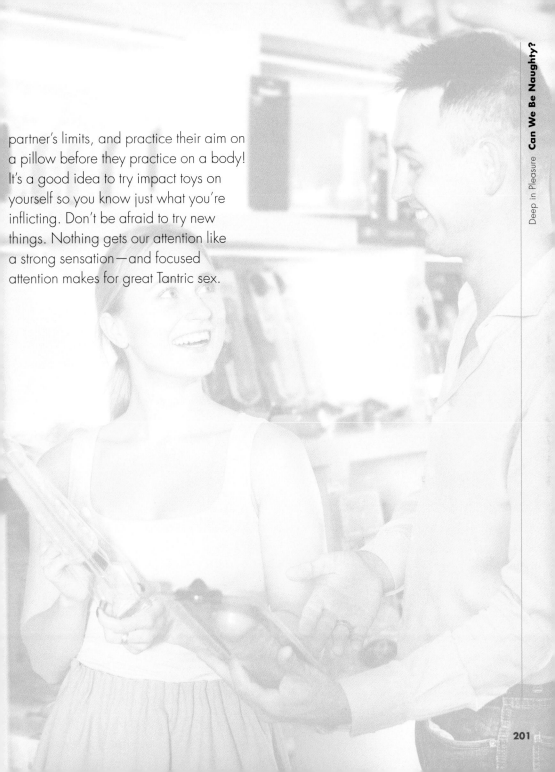

partner's limits, and practice their aim on a pillow before they practice on a body! It's a good idea to try impact toys on yourself so you know just what you're inflicting. Don't be afraid to try new things. Nothing gets our attention like a strong sensation—and focused attention makes for great Tantric sex.

RHYTHM

Sex involves thrusting—but Tantric sex involves more than just a simple up-and-down movement. There are a range of traditional thrusts, and they can make pleasure a lot more interesting. One way to keep your body alive to new sensations is to change up the rhythm of your thrusts somewhat. Here are two particularly well-established and popular techniques in the Tantric sexual tradition.

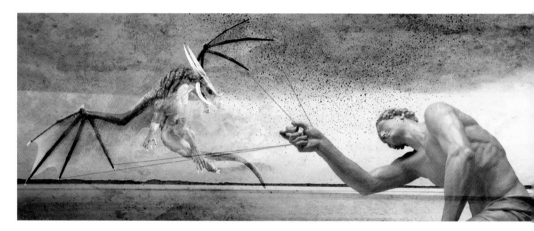

Thrusts of the Dragon

For the more advanced: nine deep thrusts followed by one shallow. For a man trying to hold off orgasm, it's more of a challenge—like the dragon, you are gathering and controlling your own power.

Thrusts of the Heron

This is a rhythm game for beginners. Start with three deep thrusts, and then make one shallow. Like the heron it is named for, you are skimming along the surface of bliss, just breaking the pattern up enough to keep things flying.

Dynamic focus

If you're trying to get into a meditative state of mind, thrusts of the phoenix really give you something to concentrate on!

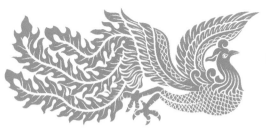

Evocative names

The traditional names of some of these rhythm techniques are evocative: let your imagination run wild.

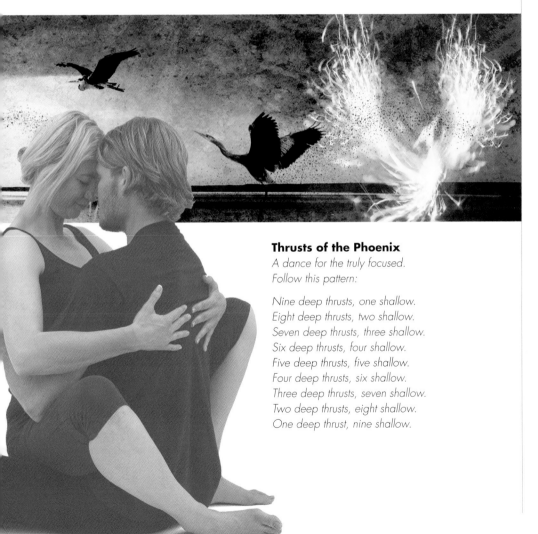

Thrusts of the Phoenix

A dance for the truly focused. Follow this pattern:

Nine deep thrusts, one shallow.
Eight deep thrusts, two shallow.
Seven deep thrusts, three shallow.
Six deep thrusts, four shallow.
Five deep thrusts, five shallow.
Four deep thrusts, six shallow.
Three deep thrusts, seven shallow.
Two deep thrusts, eight shallow.
One deep thrust, nine shallow.

STAYING SHALLOW

It can be tempting to plunge deep into your beloved, but there's a lot to be said for restraining yourself and staying near the surface of her yoni. Shallow thrusts are a lovely element to mix into your lovemaking. For one thing, they're a great way to tantalize yourselves if you're trying to prolong the moment. For another, women tend to experience more sensation at the opening of

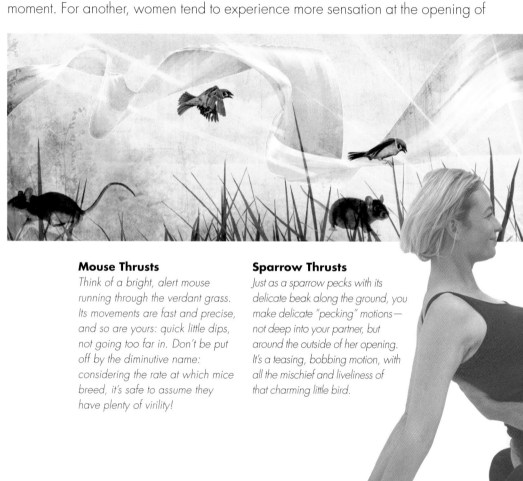

Mouse Thrusts

Think of a bright, alert mouse running through the verdant grass. Its movements are fast and precise, and so are yours: quick little dips, not going too far in. Don't be put off by the diminutive name: considering the rate at which mice breed, it's safe to assume they have plenty of virility!

Sparrow Thrusts

Just as a sparrow pecks with its delicate beak along the ground, you make delicate "pecking" motions — not deep into your partner, but around the outside of her opening. It's a teasing, bobbing motion, with all the mischief and liveliness of that charming little bird.

he vagina than deep inside, so it can be a powerful experience for her. It can also be a good technique for couples who are a wonderful fit emotionally, but maybe not the best one physically: a man with a long penis can bump a woman with a low-set cervix if he isn't careful, which often feels unpleasant, so shallow thrusts can be a gentler way to play.

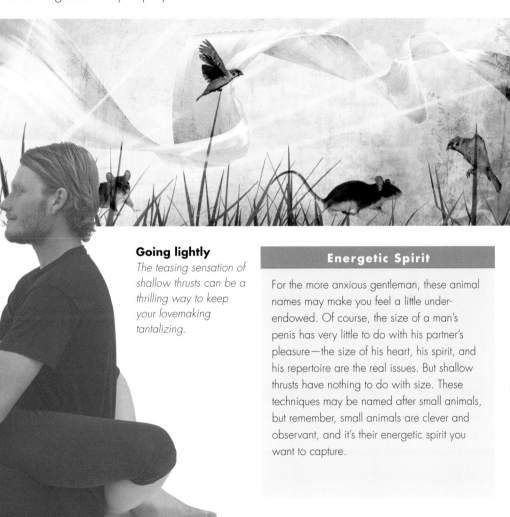

Going lightly

The teasing sensation of shallow thrusts can be a thrilling way to keep your lovemaking tantalizing.

Energetic Spirit

For the more anxious gentleman, these animal names may make you feel a little under-endowed. Of course, the size of a man's penis has very little to do with his partner's pleasure—the size of his heart, his spirit, and his repertoire are the real issues. But shallow thrusts have nothing to do with size. These techniques may be named after small animals, but remember, small animals are clever and observant, and it's their energetic spirit you want to capture.

DIVING DEEP

When you have to sink far inside your lovely partner, does that mean you have to lose control? Far from it: there are traditional thrusts that allow you to enjoy thrusting that's both deep and measured. Being as closely intertwined as you can possibly go is a wonderful experience of intimacy—an opportunity for kisses, eye gazes, and bliss. Traditional Tantric thrusts name several ways to play with such moments.

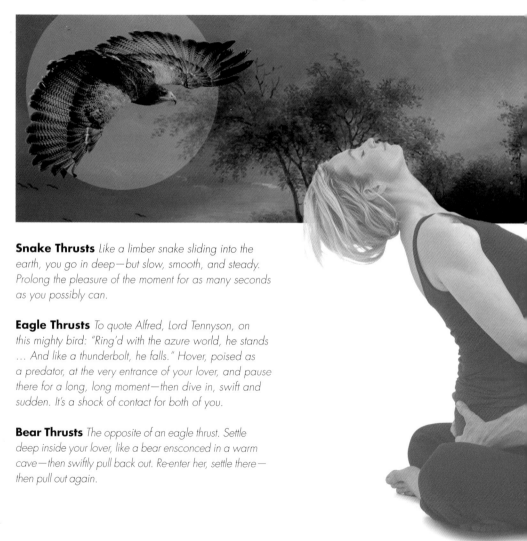

Snake Thrusts *Like a limber snake sliding into the earth, you go in deep—but slow, smooth, and steady. Prolong the pleasure of the moment for as many seconds as you possibly can.*

Eagle Thrusts *To quote Alfred, Lord Tennyson, on this mighty bird: "Ring'd with the azure world, he stands … And like a thunderbolt, he falls." Hover, poised as a predator, at the very entrance of your lover, and pause there for a long, long moment—then dive in, swift and sudden. It's a shock of contact for both of you.*

Bear Thrusts *The opposite of an eagle thrust. Settle deep inside your lover, like a bear ensconced in a warm cave—then swiftly pull back out. Re-enter her, settle there— then pull out again.*

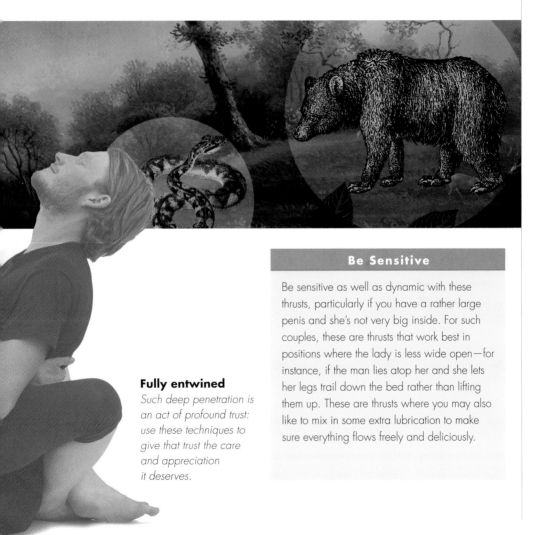

Fully entwined

Such deep penetration is an act of profound trust: use these techniques to give that trust the care and appreciation it deserves.

Be Sensitive

Be sensitive as well as dynamic with these thrusts, particularly if you have a rather large penis and she's not very big inside. For such couples, these are thrusts that work best in positions where the lady is less wide open—for instance, if the man lies atop her and she lets her legs trail down the bed rather than lifting them up. These are thrusts where you may also like to mix in some extra lubrication to make sure everything flows freely and deliciously.

207

ENERGY Sometimes you just want to go wild and stir yourselves to a pitch of frantic pleasure. When you want to prolong your pleasure, measured and skillful thrusts can be a delectable way of doing it. Tantric sex doesn't mean you're never allowed to give way to passion, though—that would be a pretty frustrating love life. To build up energy for a climactic release, try these thrusts when it's really time to let yourselves go.

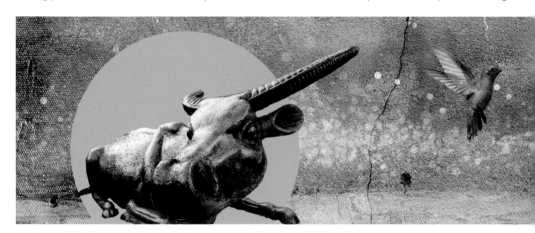

Ox Thrusts

If you want to build up a deep, inexorable rush of sensation, taking your time in a one-two rhythm, alternate one deep thrust with one shallow. Think of an ox's strong, steady stride: it doesn't rush, but nothing in the world is going to stop it in its path.

Horse Thrusts

Like a wild horse bucking, you just go for it: fast, deep, and reckless, forgetting everything but the blaze of desire. This is not a method likely to prolong your intercourse, of course, but there are moments when you just have to.

Transcendent passion

In moments of abandon, your mind can be entirely focused on the sensations of your body. Embrace such moments: within Tantric lovemaking, they too can be moments of meditation.

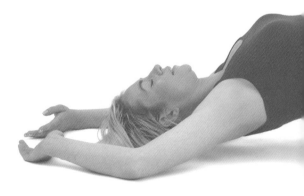

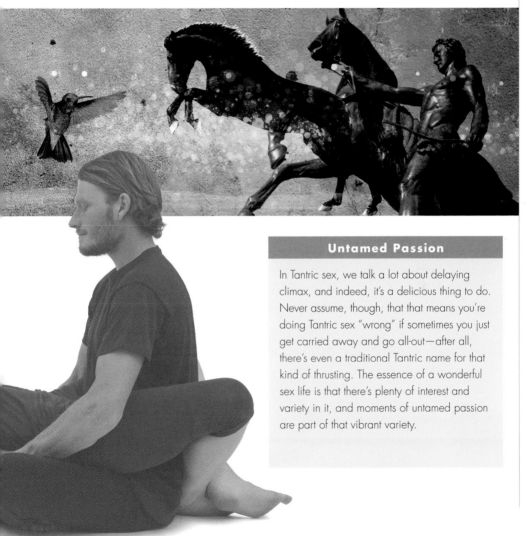

Untamed Passion

In Tantric sex, we talk a lot about delaying climax, and indeed, it's a delicious thing to do. Never assume, though, that that means you're doing Tantric sex "wrong" if sometimes you just get carried away and go all-out—after all, there's even a traditional Tantric name for that kind of thrusting. The essence of a wonderful sex life is that there's plenty of interest and variety in it, and moments of untamed passion are part of that vibrant variety.

AFTERGLOW

Lovemaking doesn't end at orgasm. Be prepared for your body to experience a come-down after that great energy release, and nurture each other. It's a common stereotype: after sex, the man rolls over and falls asleep, leaving his lonely lady-love to lie awake feeling abandoned. This is not how to relax after Tantric lovemaking. A deeply spiritual experience can leave you buzzing with energy, and perhaps experiencing strange states of consciousness that you need to play out before you can talk normally. Try resting in these peaceful positions to let the moment settle.

Finding the Balance

It is true that sex can leave a person feeling that warm, heavy-muscled glow you experience when you've just burned out a great blaze of energy. (Though this isn't confined to men, and not true of every man either.) If this applies to one of you but not the other, you'll need to find a balance—but the first place to create that balance is *before* your lovemaking, in the whole of your relationship. If the more wakeful-after-sex partner feels heard, held, and cherished outside the bedroom, a little post-coital doziness will be a much smaller problem.

Together but apart

Nestled genital-to-genital, the woman rests her head between her lover's feet, while the man rests his hands on his lover's ankles. This gives you body-to-body intimacy while creating a certain "head space," in which you can process your own feelings separately for a while before returning to more verbal communication.

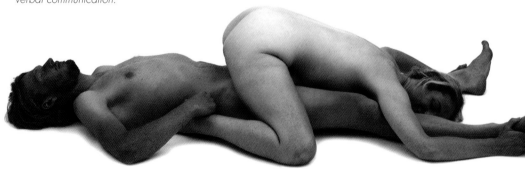

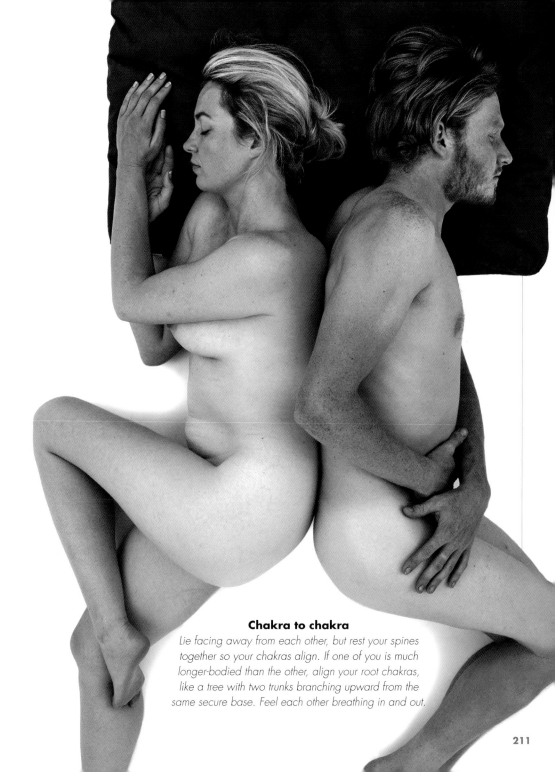

Chakra to chakra

Lie facing away from each other, but rest your spines together so your chakras align. If one of you is much longer-bodied than the other, align your root chakras, like a tree with two trunks branching upward from the same secure base. Feel each other breathing in and out.

211

Sex & Healing

Has life bruised you, spiritually or physically? Your sexual sacred space is a place of peace, acceptance, and transcendence, where you can give yourself and your partner the compassion you really need.

Sexual healing

In recent years, psychologists have been studying its effects and coming to the conclusion that the sexy old sages really did know what they were talking about—Tantric sex is, almost literally, good medicine. Expanding our definitions of orgasm and understanding of energy and pleasure has been found to help us with all sorts of issues, from moving beyond a traumatic sexual past to finding ways to physical bliss even in a severely injured body. It's amazing what you can do when you let go of your preconceptions.

We live in a society that loads all sorts of expectations onto sex, and almost all of them are wrong. If you enter your love life instead with joyful curiosity, open to letting whatever may happen happen, you are on the path to wisdom. Not to mention having a wonderful time.

Lift yourself up

The deep truth of Tantric sex is that none of us are perfect—and all of us are perfect. We are creatures of energy and flesh, deep awareness and shameless fun, all at the same time. We carry within us heavy weights: the burdens of old pain, old illusions, old inhibitions and mistakes and beliefs that hold us back. This is true. But we also carry within us the power to put down those weights and let ourselves soar.

Sex can release deep-seated emotions. If you need to have a good cry, or if you find yourself laughing for no apparent reason, or if you want nothing more than to be absolutely silent and still for a while—go for it! Listen to what your self is telling you. Release that tension. Embrace those emotions. Fill yourself with pleasure until there's no room for anything else.

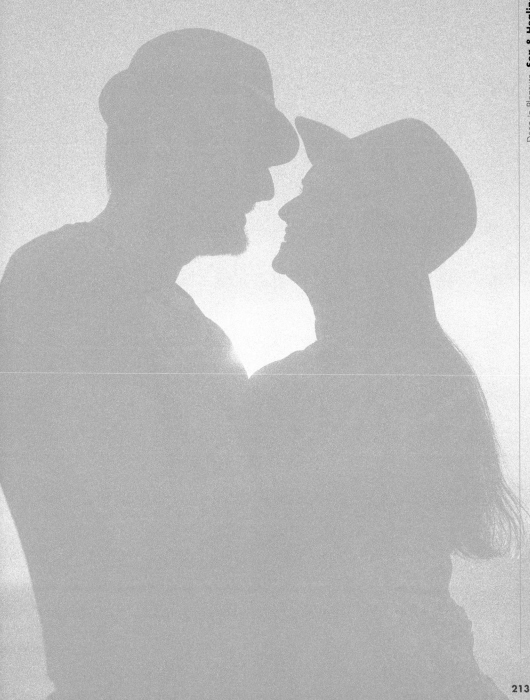

APPENDICES

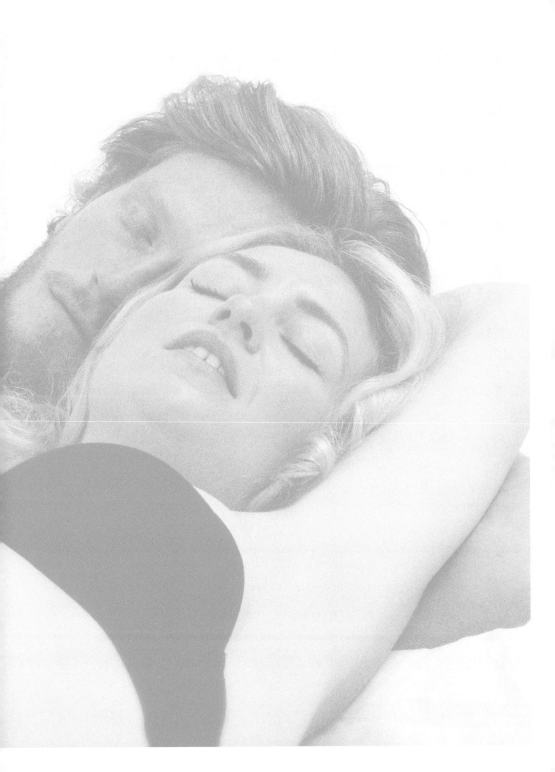

GLOSSARY

Affirmation A positive, encouraging phrase you can write or repeat to yourself in order to help you accept and feel its truth.

Bulbocavernosus muscle A muscle in the perineum (i.e. between the anus and the genitals), which can be strengthened by exercise to support more powerful orgasms and greater sexual stamina.

Chakra The seven centers of energy in our body, beginning at the base of the spine with the root chakra and rising to the top of our scalp with the crown chakra. Much of Tantric sex depends on experiencing the flow of energy through the chakras and learning to control and enjoy it.

Edging Riding the "edge" of arousal, sustaining pleasure without quite tipping over into orgasm.

Kundalini "Coiled" energy, held at the base of the spine, that can be awakened through the chakras. A concept common in both Tantric sex and yoga.

Lingam A Sanskrit-derived term for "penis." From "linga," meaning "mark," as in a mark of maleness or Shiva energy.

Loving-kindness A quality of unjudging warmth and well-wishing, toward both self and others, that underpins the spiritual journey. Many philosophies have their own term for this universal concept; "metta" is a common term in Buddhism, while the Christian "charity" also comes close.

Orgasm In Tantric sex, a release of spiritual as well as physical energy.

Meditation The practice of bringing your mind gently to focus on a single aspect of your experience or perception. Understood in both East and West to be a powerful foundation for emotional health.

Pleasure [verb] "Making love" to your partner—in the broadest sense, which is to say, using your body, your words, your feelings, and your spirit to give them delight.

Pubococcygeus muscle A hammock-like muscle that holds steady the "pelvic floor," which plays a powerful part in the muscular contractions of orgasm.

Sacred space Both a physical "space"—Tantric lovers often like to use ritual and decoration to prepare a bedroom for lovemaking—and a psychic space in which you set aside the worries of the world and dedicate yourself to the delicious moment.

Shaivism An important tradition within Hinduism that honors the deity Shiva. Tantra is believed to have originated as a branch of Shaivism.

Taoism A philosophy originating in China, which later incorporated elements of Tantra as well. Taoism emphasizes balance, naturalness, and simplicity of spirit.

Tantrika A practitioner of the Tantric way.

Thrusting In Tantric sex, the rhythm of lovemaking has many variations that can be used to refine and prolong pleasure.

Yab-Yum position A popular position for Tantric couples seeking to bond, frequently depicted in art as a symbol of masculine compassion and virtue uniting with feminine insight.

Yang "Masculine" energy, powerful and active—which can be expressed by women as well as men.

Yin "Feminine" energy, transformative and receptive—which can be expressed by men as well as women.

Yogic breathing A deep breathing exercise that can be used to help prolong pleasure and delay orgasm.

Yoni A Sanskrit word denoting the female sexual organs; "source" or "abode" are common translations.

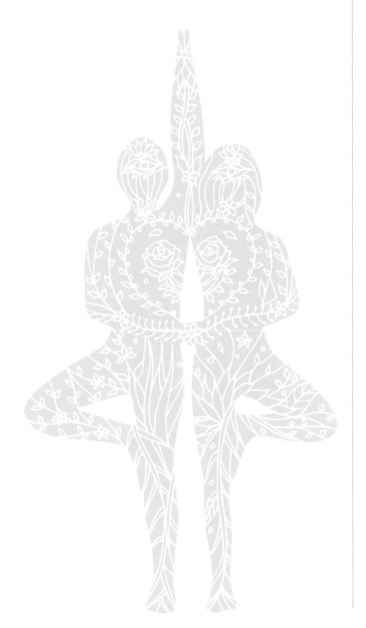

FURTHER READING

Anand, Margo. *The Art of Sexual Ecstasy: The Path of Sacred Sexuality for Western Lovers*. The Aquarian Press, 1990.

Campbell, Chris. *Tantric Sex: The Truth About Tantric Sex: The Ultimate Beginner's Guide to Sacred Sexuality Through Neotantra*. CreateSpace Independent Publishing Platform, 2015.

Carrellas, Barbara. *Urban Tantra: Sacred Sex For the Twenty-first Century*. Celestial Arts, Crown Publishing Group, Random House, 2007.

Dunne Kirby, Connie and Robert with Geraldine Ross. *Yoga for Lovers: The Way to Sensual Harmony*. Smith Gryphon Limited, 1997.

Fisher, Shubhaa. *Tantric Sex: A Beginner's Guide*. Printed in Great Britain by Amazon.

Lacroix, Nitya. *Tantric Sex: The Ancient Art of Tantra for Sensual Exploration*. Lorenz Books, 2013.

Martin, William. *The Couple's Tao Te Ching: A New Interpretation: Ancient Advice for Modern Lovers*. Marlowe and Company, Avalon Publishing Group Incorporated, 2000.

Osho. *Tantra: the Supreme Understanding*. Watkins Media, 2009.

Richardson, Diana. *The Heart of Tantric Sex*. O Books, 2003.

Riley, R. *Tantric Massage For Beginners: Discover The Best Essential Tantric Massage And Tantric Love Making Techniques!* CreateSpace Independent Publishing Platform, 2015.

Saraswati, Sunyata and Bodhi Avinasha. *Jewel in the Lotus: The Tantric Path to Higher Consciousness*. Ipsalu Publishing, 2010.

Sarita, Mahasatvaa Ma Ananda. *Divine Sexuality: The Joy of Tantra*. Findhorn Press, 2011.

Wallis, Christopher D. *Tantra Illuminated: The Philosophy, History, and Practice of a Timeless Tradition*. Mattamayura Press, 2012.

WEB SITES

About Tantra
www.about-tantra.org

Live Tantra
www.livetantra.com

Love Teachings of the Kama Sutra
www.kamasutra-sex.org

Shiva Shakti Mandalam
www.shivashakti.com

Tantra for Couples
www.tantra-essence.com/learning-tantra/tantra-for-couples

Tantra Works
www.tantraworks.com

Tantric Sex Techniques and Positions
www.sex-techniques-and-positions.com/tantra1.html

yOni
www.yoni.com

INDEX

a

afterglow 210–211
anus 127, 175

b

back massage 166–169
basic breathing meditation
    24–25
BC muscle *see*
    bulbocavernosus muscle
bear thrusts 206
belly meditation 40–41
Bhagavad Gita 10
boat pose 76–77
body acceptance 56–57
    self-acceptance exercise
    58–59
body lock technique 198
body-to-body massage 180
bound-angle pose 68–69
Brahma 12
breath control
    basic breathing meditation
    24–25
    mindful breathing 24–25
    sensual breathing meditation
    26–27
    shared breathing meditation
    104–105
    yogic breathing 63
Buddhism 13, 28–29
bulbocavernosus (BC) muscle
    78–79, 82

c

"California Tantra" 14
candles 92
canes 200
caressing meditation
    108–109
cat-cow pose 64–65
chakra dance 42–43
chakra meditation 134–135
chakra touching meditation
    170–171
chakras 36–39
circulating energy practice
    120–121
clitoral orgasms 126
clitoris 142–143
clothing 94
    see also undressing meditation
consent 96
crops 200
crown chakra 37, 39

d

dance 128–129
    chakra dance 42–43
deep thrusts 206–207
dirty jokes 111
downward-facing dog
    66–67
dragon, thrusts of the 202
dream journals 48–49
dressing the part 94

e

eagle thrusts 206
ecstasy 20–21
edging technique 62–63
ejaculation
    female 126, 173
    retrograde (injaculation) 138
emotional scars 140, 141,
    212
"emotiongasm" 54
energy
    circulating energy practice
    120–121
    drawing up 50–51, 136
    Kundalini energy 60–61
    orgasm's effect on 132–133
    see also Hollow Bamboo
equality 114–115
eye contact *see* gazing

f

fantasies 186–187
female ejaculation 126, 173
fifth chakra *see* throat chakra
fingertip massage 164–165
first chakra *see* root chakra
floggers 200
fourth chakra *see* heart chakra
frenulum 174–175

g
G-spot 126, 173
gazing during climax 154
gazing meditation 98–99
gender 116–117
     see also male and female
          selves meditation
genital massage
     for men 176–177
     for women 178–179
genitals, naming 142–143
giving pleasure 158

h
happy baby pose 74–75
harmony 88
healing 212
heart chakra 37, 38
heron, thrusts of the 202
Hinduism 10–13
Hollow Bamboo 140–141
honoring the partner 96
honoring the self 32–33
horse thrusts 208
hugging meditation 102–103

i
icons 92
impact toys 200–201
injaculation 138
Inner Alchemy (Neidan) 30
Inner Flute 140–141
inner smile meditation 30–31

k
karma 10
Kegel squeezes 80
Kundalini energy 60–61

l
Laozi (Lao Tzu) 13
laughing meditation 112–113
letting go exercise 34–35
lingam see penis
Locking the Gate 199
love letter exercise 122–123
lovers' greeting ritual 100–101
loving-kindness meditation
     28–29

m
Mahayana Buddhism 13
male and female selves
     meditation 144–145
massage
     back 166–169
     body-to-body 180
     fingertip 164–165
     genital massage for men
          176–177
     genital massage for women
          178–179
     preparing for 162–163
masturbation see self-pleasuring
meditation 22–23
     basic breathing
          meditation 24–25

belly meditation 40–41
caressing meditation
     108–109
chakra meditation
     134–135
chakra touching
     meditation 170–171
gazing meditation
     98–99
hugging meditation
     102–103
inner smile meditation
     30–31
laughing meditation
     112–113
loving-kindness meditation
     28–29
male and female selves
     meditation 144–145
sensual breathing
     meditation 26–27
shared breathing
     meditation 104–105
third-eye attunement
     118–119
third-eye meditation
     46–47
undressing meditation
     106–107
Yin–Yang 69 meditation
     184–185
metta bhavana 28–29
mindful breathing 24–25

mindfulness 23
moksha 11
mouse thrusts 204

n

naming the genitals 142–143
navel chakra 37, 38
Neidan (Inner Alchemy) 30
Neo-Tantra 14
non-ejaculatory orgasms 126

o

openness 91
orgasm
    delaying 62–63, 138,
        198–199
    effect on energy 132–133
    meaning of 54–55
    types of 126–127
ox thrusts 208

p

P-spot orgasms 126–127
paddles 200
Pangu 44
past trauma 140, 141, 212
PC/pelvic floor muscles see
    pubococcygeus muscle
penis (lingam)
    naming 142–143
    root chakra exercise for
        82–83
    understanding 174–175

phoenix, thrusts of the 203
playfulness 110–111
"pressing" technique 138
pubococcygeus (PC) muscle
    78, 79, 82, 84–85
    Kegel squeezes 80

r

receiving pleasure 158
Reich, Wilhelm 55
respect 90
retrograde ejaculation 138
rhythm techniques
    202–203
root chakra 37, 38, 79
    exercise for the penis
        82–83
    exercise for the vulva 80
    exercise with a partner
        84–85

s

sacral chakra 37, 38
sacred sexual spaces
    creating 92–93
    entering 94–95
safe sex 6, 96
scent 92, 146
second chakra see sacral
    chakra
self, honoring the 32–33
self-acceptance exercise
    58–59

self-pleasuring 32
    preparing for 128–129
    self-pleasuring exercise
        130–131
sensory awakening ritual
    146–147
sensual breathing meditation
    26–27
seventh chakra see crown
    chakra
Shakti 12–13, 116
shallow thrusts 204–205
shared breathing meditation
    104–105
Shiva 11–13, 116
silliness 110–111
sixth chakra see third-eye
    chakra
Skene's gland 173
snake thrusts 206
sparrow thrusts 204
stillness 182
straps 200

t

Tantra
    basic principles 8–9
    history 10–15
    myths debunked 18–19
Taoism 13–14, 30, 44
taste, sense of 147
teachers, finding 33
third chakra see navel chakra

third-eye attunement 118–119
third-eye chakra 37, 38
third-eye meditation 46–47
throat chakra 37, 38
thrusts
    deep 206–207
    for letting go 208–209
    rhythm of 202–203
    shallow 204–205
touch
    in massage 169
    power of 160–161
    "right or wrong" 109
    sense of 147
toys 200–201
transcendence 21
trust 91

u
undressing meditation
    106–107
Upanishads 10

v
Vedas 10
vibrators 200
Vishnu 12

w
warrior pose 72–73
watching your partner
    climax 148
    near climax 150

whips 200
wide-angle seated forward
    bend 70–71

y
Yab-Yum position 152–153
yin and yang 13–14, 44–45
    embodying 190–191
    yang-dominant positions
        192–193
    yin–yang 69 meditation
        184–185
    yin-dominant positions
        194–195
    yin and yang balanced
        positions 196
yoga exercise
    boat pose 76–77
    bound-angle pose 68–69
    cat-cow pose 64–65
    downward-facing dog
        66–67
    happy baby pose 74–75
    warrior pose 72–73
    wide-angle seated forward
        bend 70–71
yogic breathing 63
yoni
    naming 142–143
    understanding 172–173

ACKNOWLEDGMENTS

Special thanks to Anne H. for her yoga expertise and generous advice.

PICTURE ACKNOWLEDGMENTS

The publisher would like to thank the following for permission to reproduce copyright material.

Nicky Ackland-Snow 24–25, 26–27, 28–29, 30–31, 34–35, 40–41, 42–43, 46–47, 58–59, 84B, 98, 100B, 102B, 104, 106, 108, 112, 118B, 122–123, 128, 130, 144–145, 202–203, 204–205T, 206–207T, 208–209T.
Neal Grundy 9, 25, 27, 29, 30, 35, 37, 39, 40, 42, 47, 50, 58, 61, 64–77, 85, 99, 101, 103, 105, 107, 108–109, 113, 119, 120–121, 122, 127, 129, 130–131, 134–135, 137, 141, 144–145B, 149, 151, 153, 155, 162–168, 170B, 171, 176, 178, 181, 183, 185, 189–197, 199, 203B, 204–205B, 206–207B, 208–209B, 210, 211, 214–215, 219.
Peters & Zabransky 61, 62, 78, 79, 80, 82, 135T, 136, 138, 141, 172, 173, 174, 177, 179, 198,
Shutterstock/ 1933bkk: 24–25; 6348103963: 42–43; 9comeback: 203T; adike: 169; Africa Studio: 146BR; agsandrew: 58–59; Air Images: 95TR; alb_photo: 57; Potapov Alexander: 122–123; allnow: 35T; andreiuc88: 84B; andrey_l: 187; Anetlanda: 28–29; ArtemH: 55, 97; Dima Aslanian: 161; attiarndt: 11; Kitch Bain: 26–27; Alexey Belyaev: 202–203; Besjunior: 92T; Betacam-SP: 123T; Bildagentur Zoonar GmbH: 40–41; Binkski: 21; Goran Bogicevic: 115; Buslik: 46–47; Chinnapong: 40–41; Suwan CHumphone: 42–43; conrado: 42–43; cooper: 34–35; Heather A. Craig: 122–123; Alessandro Cristiano 28–29; d1sk: 34–35; Natalya Danko: 146BL; Darios: 84B; Dark Moon Pictures: 104; Dimasik_sh: 87; DM7: 202–203; Dennis W Donohue: 208–209T; dotshock: 18; dpaint: 26–27; DRogatnev: 202–203; dugdax: 93BR; DutchScenery:130; Denis Dymov: 14; Elena11: 122–123; Evannovostro: 28–29; Everett Collection: 24–25, 34–35, 98, 128; Anton Evmeshkin: 208–209T; Iakov Filimonov: 144–145, 201; franckpoupart: 102B; Christos Georghiou: 204–205T; Glass and Nature: 208–209T; Roxana Gonzalez: 42–43; goodcat: 26–27; Anne Greenwood: 26–27; Guas: 130; Antonio Guillem: 63; Gyrohype: 152; Gyvafoto: .128; Jari Hindstroem: 104; ID1974: 208–209T; IgorGolovniov: 30–31; illustrissima: 186; bogdan ionescu: 206–207T; irur: 100B; Eric Isselee: 46–47; istanbul_image_video: 30–31; Dennis Jacobsen: 202–203; Jagodka: 204–205T; K. Jensen: 98; Jianghaistudio: 26–27; Jodie Johnson: 81; JunPhoto: 40–41; K13 ART: 108; kaetana: 22; Anan Kaewkhammul: 34–35; Kanea: 144–145; Anatoliy Karlyuk: 17; Olga Korneeva: 27T; Rade Kovac: 33; Krzycho: 147T; KUCO: 58–59, 112; SUSAN LEGGETT: 122–123; LeksusTuss: 128; Alexey Lesik: 204–205T; L.F: 139; Lienhard. Illustrator: 184; LiliGraphie: 144–145; Aaron Lim: 208–209T; Ihar Linnik: 58–59; Gang Liu: 111; Madlen: 84B; Irina Maksimova: 208–209T; maodoltee: 42–43; marinatakano: 204–205T; Wiktoria Matynia: 100B; melis: 157; Nikolay Mint: 160; Luis Molinero: 95BR; Monkey Business Images: 54, 89; Evgeniya Moroz: 147B; Morphart Creation: 46–47, 58–59, 206–207T; nadtytok: 26–27; Nadya_Art: 5C; 84T, 100T, 102T, 118T, 132, 170T; nanka: 8; Bachkova Natalia: 204–205T; Roman Nerud: 122–123; Sergey Nivens: 202–203; Hein Nouwens: 58–59,100B, 206–207T; Ohishiapply:108; ohrim: 83; Byelikova Oksana: 49; oneword: 34–35; Only background: 144–145; ostill: 104; Pakhnyushchy: 204–205T; Pan_Da: 202–203; PaulTrinity: 175; photoagent: 51; Photographee.eu: 93TR, 159; photolinc: 204–205T; PhotoMediaGroup: 102B; piyaphong: 34–35; Polupoltinov: 213; Andrey_Popov: 20; prettypanny: 59TR; Sasa Prudkov: 53; Michael Rayback: 5R, 56; REDPIXEL.PL: 204–205T; Ricardo Reitmeyer: 143; Emiliano Rodriguez: 116; Benjavisa Ruangvaree: 4R, 6T, 217; Dmitriy Rybin: 28–29; Mario Saccomano: 36; Serebrennikov: 15; Denis Shevyakov: 142; Sollex 37–39; Jason Stitt: 19; StockLite: 94T; Boris Stroujko: 2; Studio DMM Photography, Designs & Art: 42–43; studiovin: 144–145; suronin: 23; SvetaZi: 117; taviphoto: 144–145; traveliving: 125; Travel Stock: 206–207T; TRyburn: 202–203; umpo: 204–205T; vadik4444: 34–35; Martins Vanags: 40–41; vasara: 44; Oleksandra Vasylenko: 24–25; velora: 46–47; vetre: 40–41; Wang Jie (Jay Wang): 40–41; wavebreakmedia: 48, 90–91, 112; WAYHOME studio: 114; Yanas: 208–209T; vladimir yermakov: 144–145; claudio zaccherini: 32; Piotr Zajda: 130; ZaZa Studio 24–25; Michal Zduniak 34–35.
Wellcome Library, London 10–11, 12, 13, 45, 133.